Directory of
Information Resources
for the
Handicapped

Directory of Information Resources for the Handicapped

by
The Staff of
Ready Reference Press

A Guide to Information Resources and Services for the Handicapped

READY REFERENCE • SANTA MONICA, CALIFORNIA

Library of Congress Cataloging in Publication Data

Ready Reference Press.
    Directory of information resources for the handicapped.

    Includes index.
    1. Handicapped—Services for—United States—Directories. 2.
Handicapped—Information services—United States—Directories. I. Title.

HV1553.R4   362.4'07   80-53529
ISBN 0-916270-28-9

TABLE OF CONTENTS

Information Resources for the Handicapped

Appendices

Part One

ADVOCACY, CONSUMER, VOLUNTARY HEALTH ORGANIZATIONS

Page

**Affiliated Leadership League of and for
    the Blind of America (ALL)**
879 Park Avenue
Baltimore, MD 21201
(301) 752-4230

Handicapping Conditions Served: Blindness.

The Organization: The Affiliated Leadership League of and for the Blind of America (ALL) is a coalition of 60 national and local membership organizations which serve the blind. The primary function of the coalition is advocacy; it testifies before congressional committees and advises Federal agencies and national private organizations on the needs and rights of blind persons. ALL's main concerns are fund-raising ethics, human and civil rights, and the utilization of qualified blind people in management positions.

Information Services: ALL publishes a bimonthly newsletter which reports on pending legislation, current hearings, new publications for the blind, and new technology. Cassettes can be obtained on loan from the organization which detail the services available from each member organization.

**Alexander Graham Bell
    Association for the Deaf**
3417 Volta Place, N.W.
Washington, DC 20007
(202) 337-5220 (Voice/TTY)

Handicapping Conditions Served: Deafness and hearing impairments.

The Organization: The Alexander Graham Bell Association for the Deaf, founded in 1890, is committed to the idea that hearing-impaired children should be afforded the opportunity to develop spoken communication through the effective use of amplified residual hearing and speechreading skills. The Association's Children's Rights Program advocates educational options for deaf children and provides consultant services for families pursuing their legal rights. Through this program, volunteers throughout the country serve as knowledgeable local resources for hearing-impaired children and their families. Special divisions within the Association's membership are: Oral Deaf Adults Section, International Parents' Organization, and American Organization for the Education of the Hearing Impaired.

Information Services: The Association publishes a journal, *Volta Review*, an annual monograph, and a newsletter. It also publishes a variety of books and audiovisual materials concerning the psychological, social, and educational implications of hearing loss. The Association sponsors an International Lecturer's Series, regional conferences, and a biennial convention.

The Association maintains a library of works of both historical and current importance in the field of deafness. A lending library of current materials is available to members.

The Association disseminates informational materials and answers inquiries from hearing-impaired persons, their families, professionals, and the general public. For additional information, contact the Manager of Information Services.

American Brittle Bone Society (ABBS)
Cherry Hill Plaza, Suite LL-3
1415 East Marlton Pike
Cherry Hill, NJ 08034
(609) 829-6212

Handicapping Conditions Served: Osteogenesis imperfecta and osteoporosis.

The Organization: The American Brittle Bone Society (ABBS) was founded in 1977 to act as an information and support group for victims of brittle bone disease, specifically osteogenesis imperfecta (congenital) and osteoporosis (degenerative, affecting adults). These are metabolic diseases which affect not only the vulnerability of bones to fracture, but may involve conditions of the heart, skin, muscles, teeth, and other organs of the body.

Information Services: ABBS provides free information to lay and professional persons about brittle bone disease and its management. A parent packet contains eight pamphlets relating to management of children with brittle bone disease and to medical needs of the child. Professional materials include brochures and reprints about osteogenesis imperfecta and osteoporosis. A periodic newsletter reports research developments and includes human interest articles.

The Society operates a hotline between 8 a.m. and 5 p.m. daily (at the above number), to provide moral support, information about management of the disease, and referrals to physicians and treatment centers. For further information, contact Mrs. Roberta DeVito, Chairman of the Board.

American Cancer Society (ACS)
777 Third Avenue
New York, NY 10017
(212) 371-2900

Handicapping Conditions Served: Cancer.

The Organization: The American Cancer Society supports research into the causes and detection of cancer and educates primary care physicians and the public to recognize the signs of cancer. ACS offers a variety of research project grants to institutions and personnel in every aspect of cancer research. The Society's public education programs emphasize the value of periodic checkups and cancer's seven warning signals and are carried out by ACS volunteers in homes, places of employment, community meetings, and through the media. Professional education programs, offered through literature, conferences, and on-site hospital visits, are designed to motivate the medical and allied professions to use the latest and best possible cancer detection, diagnostic, and patient management techniques.

ACS provides direct services to the cancer patient through its 58 state and large city divisions and 3000 county units. These services include loans of sickroom supplies, surgical dressings prepared by volunteers, and transportation to and from place of treatment. Trained volunteers, who have been treated for cancer, assist cancer patients through ACS sponsored rehabilitation programs, such as: 1) **The International Association of Laryngectomees**, which offers speech training and moral support to the laryngectomy patient (see separate entry); 2) **Reach to Recovery**, which provides counseling and special exercises for the mastectomy patient; and 3) an ostomy rehabilitation program, which gives psychological support and trains enterostomal therapists who work with patients in adjusting bodily functions to daily living. All rehabilitation programs are medically directed and supervised.

Information Services: The ACS medical library functions as a repository and clearinghouse of information on all aspects of cancer for physicians, nurses, researchers, clergymen and other professionals. Printed materials on cancer safeguards, cancer detection, smoking, statistical information, and information on unproven methods of cancer detection and treatment are available for the lay public. The Society publishes a variety of professional journals and publications. Most materials are provided free of charge. The ACS divisions and units provide general information services and referrals to area physicians, hospitals, and sources of financial assistance.

**American Coalition of Citizens
    with Disabilities (ACCD)**
1200 15th Street, N.W.
Suite 201
Washington, DC 20005
(202) 785-4265 (Voice and TTY)

Handicapping Conditions Served: All handicaps.

The Organization: The American Coalition of Citizens with Disabilities (ACCD) is comprised of 90 member agencies which represent specific handicapping conditions. The ACCD acts as a unified voice of its member organizations to support legislation for the handicapped, particularly in the areas of transportation and education. Working through and with an employment agency for the handicapped, ACCD offers job placement services for the handicapped.

Information Services: ACCD collects information about transportation problems and available special services in more than 30 states. It answers inquiries from the public about such services and about the legal rights of the handicapped. The Coalition holds educational training seminars in local communities to inform handicapped people about the educational opportunities available to them through Federal, state and local programs. Local workshops are held in advocacy training to teach the handicapped about their legal rights, how to lobby, and how to work with the media. ACCD publishes monthly and quarterly newsletters, which report on major issues of concern to the handicapped. Other publications include: *Rehabilitating America, Planning Effective Advocacy Programs*, and *Self-Help Groups in Rehabilitation*. For information, contact John Williams, Director of Public Relations.

American Council of the Blind (ACB)
Suite 506
1211 Connecticut Avenue, N.W.
Washington, DC 20036
(202) 833-1251

Handicapping Conditions Served: Blindness, visual impairments, and deaf-blindness.

The Organization: The American Council of the Blind (ACB) advocates legislation for the blind and other handicapped persons. Priority areas of advocacy include civil rights, social security and supplemental security income, national health insurance, eye research, and low vision technology. The Council has 14 national agency affiliates of the blind which support its advocacy programs. These include the Randolph Sheppard Vendors of America, a parents' organization for visually impaired parents and parents of visually impaired children, an organization of guide dog users, and vocationally oriented organizations for professionals (e.g., blind lawyers, blind secretaries, and blind computer programmers). ACB's 45 state chapters monitor state laws affecting the blind. The National office offers free direct legal assistance to groups in discrimination and benefits cases and to individuals in precedent cases.

Information Services: ACB holds periodic workshops for the blind on advocacy and legal rights. The organization has information about agencies and schools for the blind, national health insurance proposals, how to establish a credit union for the blind, electronic aids, legislation, and legal rights. It can often give advice about specific legal problems over the phone. If ACB is unable to give legal assistance, it will provide referrals to other possible sources. A monthly magazine updating developments in legislation, education, and employment is available in large print, braille, disc, or cassette. For information, contact Kathy Megivern, Staff Attorney.

American Diabetes Association (ADA)
600 Fifth Avenue
New York, NY 10020
(212) 541-4310

Handicapping Conditions Served: Diabetes mellitus.

The Organization: The American Diabetes Association is a national membership organization for professionals and lay persons, with 56 affiliates (state and large city) and 700 local chapters. ADA supports research into the cause, treatment and cure of diabetes. It sponsors professional, patient and public education programs. ADA affiliates conduct diabetes screening tests and offer youth programs, such as summer camps, parent and youth groups, and young adult discussion groups.

Information Services: ADA conducts frequent professional seminars, scientific meetings and postgraduate courses for physicians and other health personnel, and it publishes two professional journals. Patient education programs include monthly meetings, in-hospital orientations, seminars and 24-hour "hotlines." In addition to basic fact books, ADA publishes lay and professional pamphlets about diet, diabetes and its relationship to other medical problems, insulin and other drugs, travel tips, and a variety of other subjects. A bimonthly magazine, primarily for the diabetic patient, includes feature articles, reports on recent research, recipes, and affiliate activities. Affiliates provide a variety of information, especially on diet, and serve as referral sources to appropriate direct care agencies.

American Foundation for the Blind (AFB)
15 West 16th Street
New York, NY 10011
(212) 620-2000

Handicapping Conditions Served: Blindness, visual impairments, and deaf-blindness.

The Organization: The American Foundation for the Blind (AFB) was established in 1921 to help the blind and visually impaired acquire improved rehabilitation services and educational and employment opportunities, and to aid those persons in daily living activities. Through its national, regional, and legislative offices, AFB provides legislative consultation to government agencies, and advisory services to local agencies and schools involved in direct services. AFB conducts national and local surveys on psycho-social needs of the blind, and technological research leading to the design of a variety of devices which help the blind person to lead an independent life. The Foundation manufactures (or adapts) and sells more than 400 such devices, including braille watches, measuring instruments, shop tools, and braille games for adults and children. AFB records and manufactures about 400 talking books per year for the Library of Congress, National Library Service for the Blind and Physically Handicapped.

Information Services: AFB publishes a variety of general interest pamphlets and films about blindness, deaf-blindness, visual impairments, eye disorders, braille, assisting the blind, activities of daily living, travel, rehabilitation, education, devices, dog guides, and careers for people who wish to work with the blind. These public education materials are free in print form; films may be rented or purchased. Priced publications are mainly for professionals, and include materials on research, clinical practice, and instructional techniques in the areas of blindness, visual impairments, deaf-blindness, and other multihandicapped disabilities involving blindness. Listings of services such as *The Directory of Agencies Serving the Visually Handicapped in the United States* and *International Guide to Aids and Appliances for Blind and Visually Impaired Persons* are also published by the Foundation.

The *Journal of Visual Impairment and Blindness* covers research and practice reports, book reviews, and legislative and organizational news, and is published in print, braille, and recorded form. Other regular publications include the *Washington Report* and a quarterly newsletter.

AFB's M.C. Migel Memorial Library contains more than 30,000 books, periodicals, and other publications on blindness. Its services are available to lay and professional people, who may borrow materials in person or by mail.

Requests for information are responded to with the organization's publications or with individual letters when required. AFB makes referrals to service facilities, local agencies, and other insitutions, as appropriate.

American Heart Association (AHA)
7320 Greenville Avenue
Dallas, TX 75231
(214) 750-5414

Handicapping Conditions Served: Cardiovascular disorders and stroke.

The Organization: The primary concern of the American Heart Association is the reduction of premature death and disability due to cardiovascular disease. To this end, the AHA: 1) funds research on cardiovascular function and disease and stroke; 2) gathers information on all aspects of cardiovascular disease and stroke; and 3) disseminates the information to professionals and lay persons through its publication and the media.

Information Services: AHA's 2000 local affiliates act as information and referral centers. Public education and community programs focus on the early recognition, diagnosis and treatment of cardiovascular diseases. Topics include risk factors, early warning signs of heart attack and stroke, control of high blood pressure, rheumatic fever prevention, and cardiac and stroke rehabilitation. Also available to the lay person are directories of stroke clubs, acute stroke treatment centers, and cardiac rehabilitation units. Professionals can obtain printed materials on successful rehabilitation programs and facilities, exercise testing and training, and standards for testing laboratories. Journals are published for physicians and researchers, and two cardiovascular disease newsletters are printed for physicians and nurses. Publication catalogs are available from local affiliates and the national office. AHA holds professional continuing education seminars nationwide. Each AHA affiliate acts as a referral agency to direct services available in its locality, such as cardiac and stroke rehabilitation centers, dieticians, smoking cessation classes and dieting workshops. For information, contact a local AHA office.

American Lung Association (ALA)
1740 Broadway
New York, NY 10019
(212) 245-8000

Handicapping Conditions Served: Respiratory conditions.

The Organization: The American Lung Association (ALA) seeks the eradication and control of tuberculosis and chronic obstructive pulmonary diseases, including chronic bronchitis, asthma, and emphysema. It develops materials and programs of professional and public education and research in five major areas: (1) occupational health; (2) clean air conservation; (3) smoking and health; (4) pediatric pulmonary disease; and (5) adult pulmonary disease. The medical arm of the ALA, the American Thoracic Association, conducts specific research and acts as a medical advisor to the ALA and its 200 local chapters and 60 constituent (state and large city) chapters. The chapters offer some direct services, such as smoking cessation clinics and breathing improvement classes. ALA provides seed grants to young researchers, and fellowships and grants to universities.

Information Services: Printed materials, films and resource materials on emphysema, chronic bronchitis, air pollution, smoking and health, tuberculosis and other lung diseases are available free to lay and medical persons. ALA publishes monthly and quarterly professional journals and maintains nationwide lists of pulmonary rehabilitation centers, smoking cessation clinics, and Federal and national facilities and services. Local and constituent chapters maintain local directories of facilities and direct care providers, and act as lung information and referral centers. For information, contact the ALA at the above address or a local lung association listed in the telephone book.

American Parkinson Disease Association (APDA)
147 E. 50th Street
New York, NY 10022
(212) 421-5890

Handicapping Conditions Served: Parkinson's disease.

The Organization: The American Parkinson Disease Association (APDA) was founded for the purpose of providing information about the various services available to patients with Parkinson's disease and for making funds available for research in new drug therapies. It subsidizes Parkinson's disease clinics in 15 locations throughout the United States which provide treatment and act as local referral sources. The APDA awards research grants to universities and hospitals. In addition, each year a $50,000 Senior Research Fellowship is awarded to an outstanding medical researcher for three year periods, to aid in finding a cure for Parkinson's disease.

Information Services: APDA publishes four pamphlets and a quarterly newsletter for Parkinson patients and their families. The four pamphlets are: 1) *A Manual for Patients with Parkinson's Disease;* 2) *Aids Equipment and Suggestions to Help the Patient with Parkinson's Disease in the Activities of Daily Living;* 3) *Speech Problems in Parkinson's Disease;* and 4) *Home Exercises for Patients with Parkinson's Disease.*

The newsletter provides up-to-date information about new treatments, medications, and research. The national APDA keeps updated lists of treatment centers and self-help groups across the country. For patients in the New York City area, the national APDA office can refer to local physicians, equipment sources, home health care services, and transportation services. For information, contact Amy Pollard, Coordinator of Patient Services, at APDA.

American Veterans of World War II,
**   Korea, and Vietnam (AMVETS)**
1710 Rhode Island Avenue, N.W.
Washington, DC 20036
(202) 223-9550

Handicapping Conditions Served: All handicaps.

The Organization: AMVETS is a service organization for veterans, including handicapped veterans. The organization operates at national, state and local levels with 1400 local posts across the country. Its main concerns for handicapped veterans are veterans benefits—education, rehabilitation and employment—and legislation affecting the handicapped. A legislative staff in Washington keeps abreast of all new legislation affecting veterans and the handicapped, and maintains a close liaison with Congress. Individual advocacy is provided nationwide through a network of service officers located at regional offices of the Veterans Administration (VA).

Information Services: Although AMVETS is a membership organization, information and direct services are available to any veteran or dependents of veterans. AMVETS' primary effort is at the state and local levels, through service officers and accredited representatives. The officers and representatives offer counsel, information and referrals in the areas of education, rehabilitation and employment. They act as the veteran's initial contact in obtaining these benefits, and they refer him or her to the appropriate government agency. They will appeal individual cases before an agency such as the VA if a veteran fails to get his or her rightful benefits. At the post level, AMVETS members visit hospitalized veterans, to provide whatever lay assistance they can for the patient's rehabilitation. Professional referrals and information about aids, equipment and prosthetic devices can be obtained from most service officers and post representatives, but the emphasis of each local service varies. The AMVETS newsletter includes reports on passed and pending relevant legislation. For information, contact AMVETS at the above address, or an AMVETS service office at a regional VA office.

**Amyotrophic Lateral Sclerosis Society
    of America (ALSSOA)**
15300 Ventura Boulevard, Suite 315
Sherman Oaks, CA 91403
(213) 990-2151

Handicapping Conditions Served: Amyotrophic lateral sclerosis (ALS).

The Organization: ALSSOA was established in 1975 to raise funds for research, and to help ALS patients to better cope with the disease until a cure is discovered. ALSSOA carries on an extensive public information program nationwide to locate ALS patients and provide helpful information, and to educate the public concerning the disease. Research grants are made to medical centers throughout the world. In cooperation with the University of Southern California School of Medicine, ALSSOA is engaged in a demographic study of ALS with information now being prepared for publication in the Spring of 1980. The Society provides peer counseling for patients and their family members, and information to health professionals. ALSSOA is actively involved in advocacy, working with other organizations concerned with neurological disorders to increase government sponsored research.

Information Services: In addition to the quarterly newsletter, *ALSSOAN*, which reports on patient news as well as research developments and Society activities, a news bulletin, *Hotline*, is issued to members as particularly newsworthy events occur between issues of the newsletter. A wide range of pamphlets include information on patient-family services, health insurance plans, breathing exercises, communication systems and devices, emergency treatment and support systems as well as reports and evaluations of current research. Professionals in the field as well as patients and their families are encouraged to use the Society as a clearinghouse of information on the management of ALS.

Arthritis Foundation
3400 Peachtree Road, N.E.
Suite 1101
Atlanta, GA 30326
(404) 266-0795

Handicapping Conditions Served: Arthritis.

The Organization: The Arthritis Foundation is committed to finding the cause, prevention, and cure for arthritis and allied diseases. The Foundation supports 42 arthritis clinical research centers, which are involved in treatment as well as research, and awards grants and fellowships to individuals studying arthritis. As part of the Foundation's community outreach program, volunteers from its 70 chapters make home visits to confined arthritic patients, offering assistance in daily living activities and self-help devices, such as aids to open doors and jars. Many chapters organize self-help groups for arthritic patients and the parents of arthritic children.

Information Services: The Foundation disseminates information about new drugs and therapies to its chapters and to professionals in the arthritis treatment field. A variety of lay and professional pamphlets are available from the Foundation or its local chapters, including materials specifically for the primary school teacher who has an arthritic student. Chapters maintain lists of local specialists and community services for the arthritic patient and make referrals upon request. The Foundation holds national and

9

regional scientific meetings and continuing community education programs to make local physicians aware of the latest research developments.

**Association for Children with Learning
      Disabilities (ACLD)**
4156 Library Road
Pittsburgh, PA 15234
(412) 341-1515
(412) 341-8077

Handicapping Conditions Served: All learning disabilities.

The Organization: The Association for Children with Learning Disabilities is a membership organization for professionals, adults with learning disabilities, and parents of children with learning disabilities. The national ACLD office provides general information about learning disabilities, while the 787 local chapters provide referrals to physicians and treatment centers. One of the prime functions of the national ACLD is the advocacy of educational and rehabilitative legislation affecting the learning disabled. The ACLD conducts its own research into the link between juvenile delinquency and learning disabilities. With its state affiliates, ACLD works directly with school systems on early identification and diagnosis, as well as remediation in integrated specialized classroom situations. Direct services, such as parent counseling, nursery school, and day camps are provided by many of the local chapters; no direct services are available at the national level.

Information Services: Through state and national conferences, the ACLD distributes information on new technology for teaching the learning disabled. For these meetings, ACLD gathers outstanding professionals to speak and answer questions concerning the nature of learning disabilities and the education available to the learning disabled. Pamphlets and scientific reprints are available at no cost. National lists of colleges, private schools, and summer camps with facilities for the learning disabled are compiled and updated by the national organization. The ACLD newsletter covers clinical advancements and legislative developments affecting the learning disabled. A bibliography of more than 400 professional and lay publications on learning disabilities is available. For information, contact Mrs. Jean Peterson, Executive Director, at the above address.

Association for Retarded Citizens (ARC)
National Headquarters
2709 Avenue E East
Arlington, TX 76011
(817) 261-4961

Handicapping Conditions Served: Mental retardation.

The Organization: The goals of the Association for Retarded Citizens (ARC) are to prevent mental retardation, find its cures, and assist mentally retarded persons in their daily living. ARC's Research and Demonstration Institute conducts and sponsors projects to improve conditions for the mentally retarded. Areas of the Institute's concern include: 1) research studies on prevention and cure; 2) training volunteers working with the mentally retarded; 3) developing demonstration models for educational, training and residential facilities for the mentally retarded; 4) developing effective advocacy systems; and 5) furthering employment opportunities for the mentally retarded.

ARC's 1900 state and local units provide a variety of direct services to the mentally retarded, including day care centers, sheltered workshops, preschool programs and transportation services. **ARC-Youth** is a service-oriented organization for people 13 to 25 who work through their local units to offer direct assistance to mentally retarded members of their communities. ARC works on the national, state and local levels to communicate and interpret the needs of the mentally retarded to the public and to government agencies.

Information Services: ARC answers lay and professional inquiries about mental retardation through publications or by letter. The Association maintains a file of professional and lay articles, which it uses to research specific questions or to compile bibliographies. ARC's own publications are extensive and include pamphlets, monographs, books, handbooks and audiovisuals related to parenting, child development, citizen advocacy, civil rights, education, recreation, vocational rehabilitation, progress in research on prevention and cures, and prevention methods. General information pamphlets about mental retardation, Down's syndrome, and the Association and its activities are also available. ARC publishes a directory for service providers, *The Guide to Federal Benefits and Programs for Handicapped Citizens and Their Families*, which may be ordered from ARC's Government Affairs Office, 1522 K Street NW, Suite 516, Washington, DC 20005. The Association publishes newsletters devoted to local ARC projects, research and legislative activities. For information about direct services to the mentally retarded, contact a state or local ARC unit.

The Association for the Severely Handicapped (TASH)
1600 West Armory Way
Seattle, WA 98119
(206) 283-5055

Handicapping Conditions Served: Severe physical handicaps and profound mental retardation.

The Organization: Formerly the American Association for the Education of the Severely/Profoundly Handicapped, the organization was founded in 1974 in response to changes in legislation affecting handicapped persons and to the need for quality education and services for severely and profoundly handicapped individuals. As reflected in the name change, the organization has expanded its range of concerns to include all services to the severely and profoundly handicapped and is no longer limited to education. Membership includes not only parent and educators, but also lawyers, medical personnel, therapists, psychologists and social workers. Chapters are being chartered at local levels to facilitate increased involvement in local concerns. TASH stresses the importance of integration in living, working and learning environments for all handicapped persons.

Information Services: TASH publishes a quarterly journal containing articles of new research, trends and practices in services to severely and profoundly handicapped persons from birth to adulthood, and a monthly newsletter. Additional publications include four volumes of *Teaching the Severely Handicapped*, which reports on current research and innovations, and *Methods of Instruction with Severely Handicapped Students*. Books, papers, reprints from past issues of the journal and bibliographies are available on subjects such as vocational training, behavior modification, curricula and working with families. A bibliography of special interest to parents of severely handicapped children is available from TASH and includes reference materials on advocacy, recreation, and self-help skills development. On-going surveys include those on integrated public schools and parent needs.

TASH has recently organized a parent-to-parent network of communication. By maintaining lists of parents of severely and profoundly handicapped children who are involved in local parent support and advocacy groups, TASH is able to put inquirers in touch with parents with similar concerns. TASH also maintains a register of professional contact people who are available for assistance on specific problems of education, training of personnel, etc. Referrals to direct service providers, including schools, clinics and vocational rehabilitation services, are made by letter or phone.

**Asthma and Allergy Foundation
of America (AAFA)**
19 W. 44th Street
New York, NY 10036
(212) 921-9100

Handicapping Conditions Served: Asthma and allergic diseases.

The Organization: The main goal of the Asthma and Allergy Foundation of America (AAFA) is to increase knowledge of the causes of and the best treatment for asthma and allergic diseases. AAFA funds post-doctoral fellowships in the fields of asthma, allergy, and immunology. The organization was formerly called the Allergy Foundation of America.

Information Services: A medical professional answers mail and phone inquiries for general advice and resources, including regional lists of allergists and clinics, and furnishes professional speakers for public meetings. AAFA publishes a variety of lay pamphlets on types of allergies (hay fever, drug allergies, insect stings, etc.). Audiovisual materials, including a slide presentation about allergies and a film about exercises for asthmatics, may be borrowed by groups for a small handling charge. AAFA also publishes a lay newsletter covering scientific findings and the activities of its seven affiliated chapters.

Chapters provide varying services to their communities, including conducting educational meetings for the public, speaking at schools, and maintaining information hotlines. Hotline volunteers offer suggestions on reducing allergy irritants in the home, work, and school environments. Referrals are made to local allergists and to people in the community with similar allergies who have effectively dealt with their problems.

Blinded Veterans Association (BVA)
1735 DeSales Street, N.W.
Washington, DC 20036
(202) 347-4010

Handicapping Conditions Served: Blindness.

The Organization: The Blinded Veterans Association is a membership organization for veterans blinded during or after their military service. Advocacy, assistance, and fellowship are the goals of the organization. Direct services are based on the one-to-one principle that a blind veteran can most effectively motivate another blind veteran. BVA's **Field Service Program**, funded by the Veteran's Administration (VA), is carried out by field representatives, themselves blind, who visit blind veterans who have not been rehabilitated. They recommend rehabilitation centers, offer counseling in the areas of compensation, pensions, schooling, and the use of prosthetic aids and equipment, and counsel the veteran's family. BVA's **Outreach Employment Program**, funded by the Department of Labor, tries to convince employers, through public service advertising and direct contact, to give job opportunities to the blind veteran. BVA representatives assist the blind veteran by contacting prospective employers, and helping him to prepare resumes and job applications. They also offer counseling in job discrimination cases. BVA has 33 regional groups whose volunteer members help to provide the organization's direct services.

Information Services: BVA publishes a bimonthly printed newsletter available to all blind veterans. Members receive a phonograph recording of the newsletter along with the printed issue. The newsletter contains information about association matters, national legislation, technological advances, new publications, aids, and appliances, and where these can be obtained, as well as human interest features about blind veterans. For information, contact S. A. Vale, Acting Executive Director, at the above address.

Center on Human Policy
Syracuse University
216 Ostrom Avenue
Syracuse, NY 13210
(315) 423-3851

Handicapping Conditions Served: All handicaps.

The Organization: The Center on Human Policy is an advocacy and research organization committed to the rights of people with disabilities to integrated educational, vocational, rehabilitative, and residential services. The Center holds local, regional, and national workshops on rights, advocacy strategies, deinstitutionalization, and attitude change towards disabled students for regular classroom teachers. The Center also offers advice and backup assistance to individual consumers and advocacy groups.

Information Services: The Center publishes books, slides, and posters related to advocacy, teaching resources, institutional treatment of disabled persons, and integration. A catalog of publications and two brochures about the Center are available free upon request. The Center provides consumers with information regarding legal rights and strategies for change. It provides consultation to public schools and other agencies on the integration of handicapped persons into the community.

Committee to Combat Huntington's
Disease, Inc. (CCHD)
250 West 57th Street
Suite 2016
New York, NY 10019
(212) 757-0443

Handicapping Conditions Served: Huntington's disease (HD).

The Organization: Founded in 1967, the Committee to Combat Huntington's Disease (CCHD) now has 30 local chapters across the country. Goals of the organization are fourfold: identification of HD families; education of professionals and the lay public; promotion and support of basic and clinical research into the causes and cure of HD; and a patient services program, coordinated with various community services, to assist families in meeting the social, economic, and emotional problems resulting from Huntington's disease. CCHD has launched a nationwide legislative campaign for the establishment of clinics, genetics counseling and screening centers, and diagnostic and treatment centers. CCHD cooperates with researchers in ongoing studies. Varied patient services are offered at both the national and chapter levels.

Information Services: CCHD provides a wide range of materials for the education of the family, the professional, and the general public—most at no cost. In addition to a lending library of audiovisual materials designed for the professional, lay person, and the media, the Committee also has a lending library of general and scientific displays. CCHD participates in medical symposia and other educational events. An HD roster is being established which will serve as a unique source of data for researchers.

Consumers Organization for the Hearing
Impaired (COHI)
P.O. Box 166
Owings Mills, MD 21117

Handicapping Conditions Served: Hearing impairments.

The Organization: The Consumers Organization for the Hearing Impaired (COHI) was formed in December 1977 by the Washington Area Group for Hard of Hearing and the Organization for Use of the

Telephone. Its purpose is to organize the diverse groups of hearing impaired people—workers, students, professionals, homemakers, parents—to act as the national voice of the hearing impaired on consumer issues. One of the immediate objectives of the organization is to assure the presence of amplification systems in such facilities as auditoriums, university classrooms, theaters, movies and meeting rooms in public and private buildings. Long-range goals include promoting: 1) the modification of all public telephones for hearing aid wearers; 2) research in the fields of hearing disorders and hearing aids and devices; and 3) Federal and state financial assistance for rehabilitation services and aids for the hearing impaired.

Information Services: COHI has organizational and membership information, available free upon request.

Cooley's Anemia Foundation, Inc.
420 Lexington Avenue
New York, NY 10017
(212) 697-7750

Handicapping Conditions Served: Cooley's anemia.

The Organization: The Foundation is committed to eradication of this fatal genetic blood disease which occurs in Mediterranean people, and is usually identifiable in the age group 2-18 years. The organization maintains Cooley's anemia treatment centers and operates a blood program nationwide which supplies free blood to Cooley's anemia patients. It operates a patient service program to assist in securing chemotherapy, and a public education program to alert the at-risk Italian and Greek American population to the dangers of Cooley's anemia. In addition, the Foundation funds research projects here and abroad and conducts worldwide symposia on the disorder.

Information Services: The Foundation has a variety of printed material on the disorder and on how to deal with it, films and audiovisuals, and a newsletter. It publishes materials from the symposia it sponsors and articles on the research progress of grant recipients. The Foundation also maintains a speaker's bureau.

Cornelia de Lange Syndrome Foundation
136 Lassen Drive
San Bruno, CA 94066
(415) 952-5984

Handicapping Conditions Served: Cornelia de Lange syndrome.

The Organization: Established in 1977, the Foundation is working to develop a national parent support network to share information and offer moral support to families of affected children. Little is yet known about this rare genetic birth defect which retards both physical and mental development. A second major purpose of the organization is to assist researchers by identifying a large enough pool of families that meaningful genetic investigations can be conducted.

Information Services: A directory of parents and interested persons and the bimonthly newsletter, *Reaching Out*, are available from editor Sue Anthony, R.N., at the above address.

Cystic Fibrosis Foundation (CFF)
6000 Executive Boulevard, Suite 309
Rockville, MD 20852
(301) 881-9130

Handicapping Conditions Served: Cystic fibrosis (CF).

The Organization: The Foundation was established in 1955 to find the means for prevention, control, and effective treatment of this chronic degenerative disease involving the lungs, digestive organs, and other major organs of the body. Since there is as yet no cure or long term control of this most common genetic killer of children, CFF works through its 84 chapters to alert the general public to symptoms of the disease so early diagnosis and treatment may prolong life of victims. The Foundation helps fund more than 120 treatment centers, and makes grants to scientists, medical centers, and other organizations involved in research. Annual conferences are held for professionals in the field to present current research and to plan future projects and guidelines for treatment. CFF belongs to the International Cystic Fibrosis (Mucoviscidosis) Association which includes organizations from 26 countries. Advocacy and public awareness campaigns are conducted locally as well as nationally; local seminars and meetings for patients and their families are held periodically. Because of progress in diagnosis and treatment, many CF patients are living into adulthood. As a result, there is a widespread growth of young adult groups through which patients share their experiences in coping with the disease.

Information Services: For professionals, publications include a *Guide to Diagnosis and Management of Cystic Fibrosis* and the *Quarterly Annotated Reference* which contains abstracts of world medical literature on CF. Other periodicals include *Medical Update* and *Ed Alerts* for scientists and physicians. *CF Team Highlights* is a publication produced by and for service providers. Other materials have been prepared for teachers, potential employers, and health care personnel. Questions of higher education, marriage and family planning, and vocational training are addressed in a newsletter, *Young Adult Focus*, which carries news of local group activities as well as articles of special interest to young adults. Lists of publications, audiovisual and teaching materials, medical centers, and local chapters are available on request. Most information is available at no cost.

Disability Rights Center
Suite 1124
1346 Connecticut Avenue, N.W.
Washington, DC 20036
(202) 223-3304

Handicapping Conditions Served: All handicaps.

The Organization: The Disability Rights Center was established in 1976 to advocate for the rights of all disabled persons. At present, the Center is primarily involved in monitoring and seeking ways to strengthen the Federal agencies' affirmative action programs for the employment of disabled persons, as required by Section 501 of the Rehabilitation Act of 1973 and Section 403 of the Vietnam Era Veterans' Readjustment Assistance Act of 1974.

Information Services: The Center disseminates copies of research reports and proposals for change. Research into medical devices resulted in two publications: *Medical Devices and Equipment for the Disabled* and *Consumer Warranty Law: Your Rights and How to Enforce Them*. The Center is preparing a guide for attorneys and lay persons on how to enforce rights under Section 501.

Disabled American Veterans (DAV)
P.O. Box 14301
Cincinnati, OH 45214
(606) 441-7300

Handicapping Conditions Served: Service-connected disabilities of veterans of all wars, as well as special readjustment needs among Vietnam era veterans.

The Organization: The DAV was formed following World War I as a self-help group for veterans with service-connected disabilities. The 640,000-member nonprofit association exists solely to serve disabled veterans and their families. The DAV advocates and monitors legislation affecting the entire range of benefits for service-connected disabled veterans, including disability compensation, health care, pension, employment, vocational rehabilitation, death benefits, etc. Expert counseling and claims representation is provided to disabled veterans and their families at no cost by 280 DAV National Service Officers (NSOs) located in 67 cities in 49 states and Puerto Rico. DAV NSOs act as attorneys-in-fact, representing clients before the VA, Social Security Administration, Labor Department, HEW, and other government agencies. Since 1973, the DAV has sent Field Service Units to rural and suburban areas to serve veterans and families living some distance from a DAV office. The DAV Vietnam Vet Outreach Program focuses the skills of volunteer professionals on the unique readjustment needs of Vietnam era veterans, especially the post-traumatic stress disorder often referred to as Post-Vietnam Syndrome. The DAV provides disaster and emergency relief for disabled veterans and scholarships for children of needy disabled veterans. It also advocates local employment programs and removal of architectural and other barriers to the handicapped.

Information Services: A monthly news magazine covers veterans' benefits, including VA health care and veterans' legislation. General inquiries concerning rights and benefits earned by disabled veterans should be sent to the above address. Requests for assistance with benefit claims should be sent to DAV National Service Headquarters, 807 Maine Avenue, S.W., Washington, DC 20024. DAV services are provided at no cost to veterans and their families.

Down's Syndrome Congress
Penny Schimpler, Corresponding Secretary
706 S. Bunn Street
Bloomington, IL 61701
Home: (309) 829-8509
Work: (309) 827-6107

Handicapping Conditions Served: Down's syndrome.

The Organization: Formed in 1974 by a group of parents and professionals who were members of the National Association for Retarded Citizens, the Congress now has more than 70 chapters of volunteers in the U.S., Canada, and Mexico. These members share their experience with other parents, physicians and educators, and work for public awareness and acceptance of this population. An annual convention and a 10-issue newsletter keep the membership informed of new medical, legislative and educational developments.

Information Services: At local levels, members seek out parents of infants with Down's syndrome to put them in touch with the family support network and to encourage and instruct them in early home educational methods to help these infants develop their learning potentials. A brochure and fact sheets describing Down's syndrome, information on the organization and on funding of research, a revised bibliography of materials relating to the disability, and a newsletter, *Down's Syndrome News*, are available from the secretary, who also answers inquiries and makes referrals to local chapters or resource people.

16

Dysautonomia Foundation, Inc.
370 Lexington Avenue
New York, NY 10017
(212) 889-0300

Handicapping Conditions Served: Familial Dysautonomia.

The Organization: Established in 1951 by parents of afflicted children, the Foundation now has 14 chapters in the U.S., Canada, and Israel which raise funds for research into dysautonomia and provide information on this genetic disorder to the medical community and patients' families. The condition affects the autonomic (involuntary) nervous system and to a lesser extent the central nervous system, with a variety of symptoms. Confined to children of Eastern European Jewish ancestry, Familial Dysautonomia is a rare and often misdiagnosed disease; therefore education of pediatricians and parents in early detections and care is a primary concern. The Foundation maintains a **Dysautonomia Treatment and Evaluation Center** at New York University Medical Center for the benefit of patients and their physicians. A national medical symposium on the disorder is held annually for research scientists, clinicians and health care professionals.

Information Services: A variety of printed material is available without cost, including handbooks on nursing and family care of patients, reprints of articles from both professional and lay publications, bibliographies, fact sheets and brochures on the disease, and a public education film, "Without Tears." Lists of local chapters, schools and camps familiar with the disorder, and names of physicians experienced in treating patients with the disorder can also be requested.

Epilepsy Foundation of American (EFA)
1828 L Street, N.W.
Washington, DC 20036
(202) 293-2930

Handicapping Conditions Served: Epilepsy and seizure disorders.

The Organization: The Epilepsy Foundation of America (EFA), with its 100 affiliated chapters and 60 local information and referral services, is involved in advocacy and a wide variety of services and programs for the person with epilepsy. EFA sponsors a number of special projects, such as: 1) *School Alert*—designed to improve school environments for children with epilepsy by providing materials to help students, teachers and other school personnel understand the condition better; 2) *Community Alert*—information for the community official, including police, firefighters, ambulance personnel, and others on what to do for a person having a seizure; 3) *Self-Help*—involves people gaining strength and encouragement from the sharing of common experiences and the undertaking of common objectives; 4) *Training and Placement Service*—provides training and placement service to young people; and 5) *Seed-Grant*—designed to get promising research projects started and promising people into the field of epilepsy research. Such special projects are provided on a demonstration basis in the hopes that they will be supported by or incorporated into existing community agencies.

Information Services: EFA provides information on epilepsy and its consequences to any person or group requesting it. Areas include: 1) information on epilepsy for the patient, his family and friends; 2) educational material to individuals and groups dealing with people with seizure disorders; 3) information on employment, including vocational rehabilitation and training, rights, hiring and insurance regulations, special programs, and the particular needs of some people with epilepsy whose seizures are not fully controlled; 4) specific information on the rights of persons with epilepsy as guaranteed by Federal and state statutes; 5) housing information (mostly about discrimination and alternative living arrangements, such as group homes); 6) transportation information, including Federal and state driving regulations; 7) health service information, including prevention, diagnosis, treatment, rehabilitation, and maintenance; 8) information on economic, social and psychological services, such as disability benefits and supplemental security income, recreational services, and individual and group counseling programs; 9) information on

17

the latest research into the causes, treatment and prevention of seizures; and 10) information on Federal and state programs that affect people with epilepsy. Many local chapters offer similar informational services. Some are affiliated with epilepsy clinics or work closely with them. A directory of epilepsy clinics is available from EFA. EFA publishes pamphlets, reprints, books, cassettes, slides, films and a monthly newsletter.

Friedrich's Ataxia Group in America, Ind. (FAGA)
P.O. Box 11116
Oakland, CA 94611

Handicapping Conditions Served: Friedreich's ataxia.

The Organization: A voluntary organization of patients and other interested persons, FAGA was founded in 1970 to act as a clearinghouse of information on this rare genetic neuromuscular disorder. FAGA is active in fund raising efforts to support research into the causes and treatments of the disorder. Actual treatment of patients and orthopedic appliances are provided by Muscular Dystrophy Association clinics.

Information Services: The organization publishes a quarterly newsletter and a brochure, *What Is Friedreich's Ataxia*? Membership information may be obtained by writing to the organization.

Human Growth Foundation (HGF)
4930 West 77th Street
Minneapolis, MN 55435
(612) 831-2780

Handicapping Conditions Served: Growth retardation.

The Organization: The members of the Human Growth Foundation (HGF) are parents of children with severe physical growth problems, and physicians and scientists specializing in the field of growth retardation. The Foundation supports research in endocrinology, and working with the National Pituitary Agency, tries to secure pituitary glands through donor pledges. Pituitary glands are the only source of human growth hormone (HGH), which is often used in the treatment of growth retardation. Twenty local chapters of HGF provide opportunities for parents to share problems associated with their short-statured children.

Information Services: The national and local organizations provide parent and public educational materials about growth problems. Pamphlets on specific growth disorders, such as Turner's syndrome and achondroplasia, are available as are general information brochures on problems in parenting a growth-retarded child, scientific developments, foundation information, and how to become a pituitary gland donor. HGF refers to physicians who specialize in growth retardation.

International Association of Laryngectomees (IAL)
American Cancer Society (ACS)
777 Third Avenue
New York, NY 10017
(212) 371-2900

Handicapping Conditions Served: Laryngectomy.

The Organization: The International Association of Laryngectomees (those whose larynxes have been surgically removed) is a coordinating organization of more than 280 laryngectomee clubs located in the

U.S. and abroad. It is financially sponsored by the American Cancer Society (see separate entry). IAL club members are larnygectomees and speech therapists who provide rehabilitation (esophogeal speech training), motivation and moral support to newly laryngectomized patients on a volunteer basis.

Information Services: IAL publishes brochures and fact sheets about speech training, speech devices, medical, nursing and family care of the laryngectomee, psychological problems of the laryngectomee, first aid and vocational adjustment problems. Bibliographies, reprints and professional papers are available on similar subjects of interest to the patient, his family and professionals. IAL's major publications include: 1) *Annual Directory*—listing member clubs, meeting dates and place, availability of speech instruction, and local sources of supplies—from bibs to artificial larynxes to medical, rehabilitation and teaching films; 2) *Laryngectomized Speaker's Source Book*—includes information on cancer of the larynx, problems faced by laryngectomees, speech of the laryngectomee, speaking tips, rehabilitation needs, and information about the IAL; and 3) *Registry of Laryngectomized Instructors of Esophageal Speech*.

A bimonthly newsletter reports on club activities. All materials may be obtained from ACS national or local offices. IAL refers inquirers to speech therapists, but does not make medical referrals.

**International Association of Parents
 of the Deaf (IAPD)
814 Thayer Avenue
Silver Spring, MD 20910
(301) 585-5400**

Handicapping Conditions Served: Deafness, hearing impairments, and deaf-blindness.

The Organization: The International Association of Parents of the Deaf (LAPD) is a membership organization operated in alliance with the National Association of the Deaf. It acts as a clearinghouse for the exchange of information among parents of the deaf and between parents of the deaf and professionals. A "Key Network" of parents across the country contact and motivate others when action must be taken on important issues such as legislation. IAPD has 32 affiliated groups in the U.S., Canada, and Iran.

Information Services: IAPD provides general information about deafness and raising deaf children including deaf-blind children to all inquirers at no cost. It refers new inquirers to other parents of deaf children in their own geographical areas, so that they can share their concerns and experiences. IAPD provides speakers to its affiliated groups for workshops and seminars. The organization also publishes a bimonthly newsletter, available to members, which includes information about developments in education, legislation, and aids for deaf children.

**Jewish Guild for the Blind (JGB)
15 West 65th Street
New York, NY 10023
(212) 595-2000**

Handicapping Conditions Served: Blindness and visual impairments.

The Organization: The Jewish Guild for the Blind (JGB) offers a wide range of services to blind and visually impaired persons and their families, without regard to religion, race or age. Direct services include: 1) rehabilitation in the areas of daily living activities and orientation and mobility; 2) vocational counseling, specialized job training and job placement; 3) jobs in sheltered workshops (bagging, collating, sewing, etc.); 4) workshops and courses in arts, crafts and music for all age groups; 5) mental health services including a psychiatric clinic, a school for multihandicapped children, a day treatment program and a hostel, both for multihandicapped young adults. A Home for Aged Blind with round-the-clock nursing and medical care is an affiliate of the Guild. JGB's clients are charged for services according to their ability to pay. The Guild offers field training experience to graduate students of social work, vocational rehabilitation, and special education.

Information Services: JGB is a major source of free current literature recordings for blind and disabled persons. More than 400 best selling books have been recorded by volunteers and the Guild distributes more than 120,000 cassettes yearly in the U.S. and abroad. A pamphlet, *Why?*, reporting the findings of a JGB study on why most people with visual impairments do not seek immediate skilled assistance in meeting the problems of sight limitation, is available free from the Guild.

Joseph P. Kennedy, Jr. Foundation
1701 K Street, N.W., Suite 205
Washington, DC 20006
(202) 331-1731

Handicapping Conditions Served: Mental retardation.

The Organization: Established in 1946, the Foundation's purpose is to raise public awareness of medical ethical problems and to improve the quality of life for the mentally retarded. To these ends the Foundation has funded research and clinical treatment centers at nine universities, instituted two centers for the study of medical ethics at Georgetown University and Harvard, underwritten fellowships in medical and nursing education for postgraduate study of medical ethics, and developed recreational programs including internships, family play programs, and the international Special Olympics Program for the mentally retarded. Proposals for innovative demonstration models from agencies or individuals are considered for funding. Extensive public awareness campaigns are carried on through the media to improve understanding and acceptance of this population.

Information Services: Brochures describing the Special Olympics Program, Let's Play to Grow Program for families, fellowships in medical ethics for nursing faculty and post-residency M.D.s, and recreational internships for the mentally retarded are available from the Foundation office. Films on the Special Olympics are available for TV or group use. Another group of films produced for education of health and other professionals includes such titles as "The Right to Survive," "The Right to Let Die," "The Right to Reproduce," and a new film, "Becky: The Value of a Life." There is a small rental or purchase fee charged for films; other information is free.

Junior National Association
of the Deaf (Jr. NAD)
Gallaudet College
Washington, DC 20002
(202) 651-5000 (Voice)
(202) 651-5104 (TTY)

Handicapping Conditions Served: Deafness.

The Organization: Established in 1960 to develop leaders among young deaf students, Jr. NAD has 82 chapters in schools and programs at secondary and post secondary levels throughout the country. Local, regional and national conferences are sponsored annually, and summer camp programs for students 10-14 and 15-20 are held each year. Awards for achievement in athletics, scholarship, writing, art and citizenship are given to encourage leadership skills.

Information Services: A quarterly magazine, *The Junior Deaf American*, and brochures on summer camp, the Jr. NAD, school selection and leadership are available from the national office.

Juvenile Diabetes Foundation (JDF)
23 E. 26th Street
New York, NY 10010
(212) 889-7575

Handicapping Conditions Served: Diabetes mellitus.

The Organization: This organization's primary objective is to support and fund research on the treatment and cure of diabetes—mainly juvenile diabetes (also called insulin-dependent diabetes), which has its usual onset from infancy to the late thirties. JDF awards grants and fellowships for specific research projects in diabetes and related areas. It sponsors national media campaigns to inform the public about diabetes and to raise funds for research. JDF's 115 local chapters provide parent to parent counseling and self help groups for newly diagnosed diabetics and their families.

Information Services: JDF publishes free pamphlets and fact sheets about diabetes and insulin for the lay person. They include such titles as: *What You Should Know About Juvenile Diabetes; Parent to Parent; Babies with Diabetes; Juvenile Diabetes Isn't Just for Kids: Having Children . . . A Guide for the Diabetic Woman;* and *What You Should Know About Insulin.* A newsletter, *Dimensions in Diabetes*, is published for JDF's members. Local chapters hold public education meetings, maintain speaker bureaus, and provide referral to medical specialists and educational programs offered by hospitals and health departments. Some chapters have an information hot-line.

Leukemia Society of America
800 Second Avenue
New York, NY 10017
(212) 573-8484

Handicapping Conditions Served: Leukemia, the lymphomas, and Hodgkin's disease.

The Organization: The objectives of the Leukemia Society of America are to find cures for leukemia, the lymphomas, and Hodgkin's desease, and to provide supplementary financial assistance to persons afflicted with those diseases. Research funds are provided to individuals investigating aspects of leukemia and related diseases. The Society's 52 chapters administer patient aid programs, whereby outpatients can receive up to $600 per year for drugs, lab fees, blood transfusions, and transportation.

Information Services: The Society publishes general information pamphlets about leukemia, Hodgkin's disease, and the lymphomas. Audiovisual materials on what leukemia is and how persons may be affected by it are available to schools and community groups. For the professional, chapters offer symposia in conjunction with local medical facilities which emphasize new developments in treatment and maintenance. Hospital visits can be arranged for medical students, so that they have the opportunity to observe patients and discuss particular cases with specialists. The Society publishes academic papers delivered by leading specialists at an international symposium held every two years. As a service to the professional and academic community, the Society maintains a bibliography of research conducted by other organizations and has a library of books and journals on leukemia and related diseases. The Society refers inquirers to leukemia centers throughout the world, and chapters provide information on possible sources of local financial aid.

Little People of America (LPA)
P.O. Box 126
Owatonna, MN 55060
(507) 451-1320

Handicapping Conditions Served: Dwarfism.

The Organization: Little People of America (LPA) was established in 1957 as a nationwide organization for dwarfs to provide fellowship, an interchange of ideas, solutions to the problems unique to the little person, and moral support. A special membership division provides opportunities for information exchange and group support to parents of dwarfed children. Twelve district directors coordinate local activities, regional and local meetings, and informal local gatherings; LPA conducts national meetings annually. LPA works closely with adoption agencies throughout the U.S., attempting to place dwarfed children in the homes of dwarfed parents. In 1968, LPA established a foundation to raise funds for vocational training of little people and medical and scientific research on the causes and possible treatment of dwarfism.

Information Services: In addition to an organizational newsletter, LPA distributes printed materials on equipment and aids, clothing, and social and vocational adjustment. Information is particularly strong in the area of driving aids. *My Child is a Dwarf* is a pamphlet of special interest to parents. LPA's medical board is used as a referral network to respond to medically-related inquiries; general inquiries are sent to district directors for responses.

Lupus Foundation of America
Virginia Masters, Secretary
4434 Covington Highway
Decatur, GA 30035
(404) 289-7453

Handicapping Conditions Served: Systemic lupus erythematosus.

The Organization: Incorporated in 1977, the Foundation is a federation of 108 chapters, many of which have been in existence for a number of years. Chapters vary in size and scope of activities; some offer educational programs to nursing schools, hospital staffs and other organizations while others fund fellowships and research grants to physicians who specialize in treatment of lupus. The chapters conduct monthly open meetings with physicians, and publish newsletters and articles to alert physicians as well as the public to the symptoms of this often misdiagnosed disease.

Information Services: Bibliographies for professionals and patients, article reprints, and pamphlets explaining the disease and treatment are available. Most information is free; a nominal charge is made for selected pamphlets and books. Information, referral lists of physicians experienced in treating lupus, and lists of local chapters may be requested from the secretary of the Foundation.

Mainstream, Inc.
1200 15th Street, N.W.
Washington, DC 20005
(202) 833-1136

Handicapping Conditions Served: All handicaps.

The Organization: Mainstream, Inc., began in July 1975 as a nonprofit tax-exempt organization whose sole purpose was to assist in the mainstreaming of the handicapped. With a Board of Directors representing industry, labor, health, education and the media, the organization works with each sector of society affected by the Rehabilitation Act to facilitate mainstreaming. The organization serves as a bridge between those who must comply with government regulations, those who enforce them, and those who are protected by them. Mainstream, Inc., sees itself as a catalyst for change in attitudes of people about the handicapped and the handicapped about themselves, and it helps to develop seminar and consultation programs on employment, accessibility and the rights of handicapped persons for interested groups.

Information Services: Anyone who has questions about legislation concerning the handicapped can find the answers by calling **Mainstream on Call**, a hotline service for corporations, educators, service providers, and the general public. This free service is available Monday through Friday 9 a.m. to 5 p.m., by calling (800) 424-8089. In addition, Mainstream publishes a free bimonthly newsletter, *In the Mainstream*, on affirmative action for the handicapped.

**March of Dimes Birth Defects
    Foundation
1275 Mamaroneck Avenue
White Plains, NY 10605
(914) 428-7100**

Handicapping Conditions Served: Congenital defects and genetic disorders.

The Organization: To achieve its goals of preventing birth defects, the March of Dimes Birth Defects Foundation funds programs in basic and clinical research, (including reproduction hazards), medical services, professional and public education, and community services. Medical services have funded 85 clinical centers in the U.S. which practice genetic medicine and counseling. In 1980, the March of Dimes plans funding at over $2 million for these genetic programs. Satellite clinics provide genetic services for areas with limited medical resources. The MOD funds intensive care services for sick newborns and follow-up studies of these infants after discharge. Emphasis now is being placed on early diagnosis and treatment of pregnant women with high risk conditions, particularly adolescents. Outreach clinics are being started in communities where prenatal care is unavailable.

Information Services: The March of Dimes funds programs through schools, churches, hospitals and other institutions to inform and motivate prospective parents and the general public to do all they can to protect maternal and newborn health. Materials include educational series, curricula, filmstrips, printed materials, films, documentaries for television, and public service announcements.

Through its Medical Education Publications Program, the March of Dimes transmits the latest scientific findings—in original articles and journal reprints—on birth defects to schools of medicine and nursing, university hospitals, medical centers, physicians, nurses and other health professionals. Also included in the publications program are: 1) the *International Directory of Genetic Services*, a listing of medical centers that provide genetic counseling and analyses of special genetic conditions; 2) the *Birth Defects Atlas and Compendium*, which standardizes names and descriptions of 1,005 congenital anomalies, in four languages, and 3) *Syndrome Identification*, an international journal of undiagnosable cases sent in by physicians from around the world.

The MOD will serve as a clearinghouse for the exchange of incidence data generated in birth defect monitoring programs in 14 countries.

The **Birth Defects Information System (BDIS)** is a computerized data base on birth defects for clinical and research uses. A summary of all known medical information about more than 1,000 of the known birth defects is presently in the computer, and data gathering on the remaining known defects is in progress. BDIS will gradually be phased into medical centers after clinical testing confirms that computerized data can assist physicians in recognizing and diagnosing birth defects. The system is connected on the TYMNET international telecommunications network, which permits access to the system through a local telephone call from most major cities in the U.S. and Europe. BDIS is operated by the **Center for Birth Defects Information Services**, which was established in early 1978 by Tufts-New England Medical Center and the National Foundation as a joint venture of these two organizations. Uses of the system include answering parents' questions (usually posed for them by a genetic counselor); assisting doctors with diagnosis; recognizing occurrences of new birth defects; printing and updating the *Birth Defects Atlas and Compendium*; training medical students by teaching diagnostic procedures; and acting as an early warning system for unusual incidence or types of birth defects, and as an aid to research on possible causes of birth defects.

23

Mental Health Association (MHA)
1800 North Kent Street
Arlington, VA 22209
(703) 528-6405

Handicapping Conditions Served: Mental and emotional disorders.

The Organization: Formerly the National Association for Mental Health, the MHA adopted its present name in 1976. Primarily an advocacy and public education organization, MHA and its 850 local chapters work for legislation affecting the rights and treatment of the mentally ill. On occasion MHA will engage in litigation, where a test case seems warranted, on such issues as regulation of electroconvulsive therapy, patients' rights to refuse drugs, or rights to counsel during commitment hearings. MHA works for improved community based treatment facilities to replace outmoded state hospitals, and it carries on public awareness campaigns to effect changes in neighborhood and business community attitudes toward recovered mental patients.

Information Services: An extensive publications list includes such titles for patient and family as *Helping the Mental Patient at Home, Civil Rights of Mental Patients,* and *What Every Child Needs for Good Mental Health.* Pamphlets for professionals include *Mental Health Education* and *On Understanding Depression.* Of interest to the general public are such publications as *How to Deal With Your Tensions, Depression: What You Should Know About It,* and *When Things Go Wrong, What Can You Do?* Information on services, insurance, research, employment, legislation and litigation, careers in mental health, rehabilitation, drug abuse and citizen activism is also available, as well as MHA position statements on topics ranging from abortion to psychosurgery. A bimonthly newsletter, *In Touch,* informs members of news in the mental health field. Films and other educational materials are available for one-day rentals; a catalog will be sent on request. Inquiries and referrals for direct service are handled by local chapters as well as the national office.

Mental Health Law Project (MHLP)
1220 19th Street, N.W.
Suite 300
Washington, DC 20036
(202) 467-5730

Handicapping Conditions Served: Mental and emotional disorders and developmental disabilities, whether actual or handicapping as a result of labeling.

The Organization: Formed in 1972 as a nonprofit public interest organization, the Project is dedicated to law reform advocacy on behalf of people labeled mentally or developmentally disabled. Test case litigation is used to define, establish, and implement the rights of such persons. Landmark judicial decisions are followed with policy advocacy at the Federal level. Priority issues include procedural protections for people subject to civil commitment; guardianship; administration of intrusive, hazardous, or experimental treatment (for example, psychoactive drugs, electro-convulsive therapy, sterilization, etc.); creation of suitable residental facilities, and provision of appropriate health and social services in the community; and enforcement of legislation which provides services and protection for discrimina-tion. MHLP offers clinical training internships for law and social work students through the Center for Law and Social Policy. Regional training conferences on mental disability law are co-sponsored with the Practicing Law Institute. Assistance in drafting legislative models and advice on legal strategies for clients appearing before administrative agencies and legislative bodies is available; when appropriate, MHLP will represent protection and advocacy organizations before Federal agencies.

Information Services: MHLP offers backup assistance to attorneys and other advocates representing mentally handicapped clients. These services include model pleadings, legal citations and technical references, discussion of strategies, and comments on pleadings, draft legislation/regulations, assistance in using experts, provision of articles, memoranda, bibliographies, etc. In answer to inquiries from professionals and other interested persons, MHLP supplies general information about legal rights and makes referrals to attorneys. Publications include *Basic Rights of the Mentally Handicapped*, a consumer handbook; *Legal Rights of the Mentally Handicapped*, a three volume course book which includes technical information about mental health and retardation issues, case law and legal analysis; and other books and reprints of articles by staff attorneys. The *MHLP Summary of Activities* reports periodically on current litigation and issues of concern. There is no charge for most information. A contribution is invited for receipt of the periodical, and reimbursement is asked for duplication and mailing of legal papers and other bulky documents.

MPS Society
552 Central Avenue
Bethpage, NY 11714
(516) 433-4410

Handicapping Conditions Served: Mucopolysaccharidoses (MPS) and mucolipidoses (ML).

The Organization: The MPS Society was founded in 1974 by parents of children with MPS or ML, types of rare, hereditary, enzyme deficiency diseases, which range in severity from strictly bone and joint involvement to complications in all organ systems. The Society's membership includes families and professionals, such as doctors, teachers, and social workers who work directly with families.

Information Services: The Society shares information about the management of children with MPS and ML, and about options to institutionalization through putting families with similarly affected children in touch with each other. Medical specialists contribute scientific information to the Society's newsletter, which also contains book reviews and organizational information, but is available to members only. The Society holds four meetings per year in various locations, at which professionals and families discuss problems of treatment and management. The national office refers families to treatment centers and physicians for specific problems.

Muscular Dystrophy Association (MDA)
810 Seventh Avenue
New York, NY 10019
(212) 586-0808

Handicapping Conditions Served: Muscular dystrophy and associated neuromuscular disorders.

The Organization: The Muscular Dystrophy Association (MDA) supports research into neuromuscular disorders. It also provides medical care and other direct services free to muscular dystrophy patients through its 217 clinics and more than 200 local chapters. MDA clinics provide diagnosis, physical therapy, medical and social counseling, and in some cases serve as clinical research centers. MDA chapters provide payment for services, including: physical, occupational, and respiratory therapies; orthopedic equipment; respiratory equipment; transportation; and flu shots. The chapters also sponsor recreational activities, such as summer camps, picnics, and outings. Some chapters organize self-help groups for muscular dystrophy patients and their families.

Information Services: MDA publishes brochures and audiovisual materials about neuromuscular diseases. Its bimonthly newsletter covers progress in research, legislation, and various MDA supported programs. A quarterly patient service publication addresses a specific topic in each issue. It offers practical suggestions on such topics as education, aids, and clothing. Publications are free and available from the MDA or its chapters, many of which publish additional informative materials. Local chapters hold patient seminars which focus on available community, financial, educational, and psychological programs. They also hold professional seminars on diagnosis, clinical management, and research. Local chapters serve as referral sources for clinics, outlets for aids and prosthetic devices, home health care providers, and vocational rehabilitation centers. For information, contact the Directory of Patient and Community Services at the above address.

Myasthenia Gravis Foundation
15 East 26th Street
New York, NY 10010
(212) 889-8157

Handicapping Conditions Served: Myasthenia gravis.

The Organization: Myasthenia gravis is a frequently misdiagnosed disease, and this Foundation was formed to fund research on the cause and cure of the disorder. In an effort to prevent misdiagnosis, promote public awareness and early detection, and publicize recent treatments, the Myasthenia Gravis Foundation offers educational services to professionals and the public. The 53 chapters and branches of the Foundation offer patient support through clinics in local hospitals, which provide both outpatient and inpatient medical care as well as chapter meetings, pill banks, hot lines, and information and referral services. Annual research grants and postdoctoral fellowships are awarded to physicians. The Foundation sponsors annual scientific meetings and international symposia every five years for medical researchers; proceedings are published.

Information Services: Direct inquiries are answered and referrals made by the local chapters as well as the Foundation headquarters. Counseling, pamphlets, and information on low cost drug banks, clinics, and recent research are available from the chapters. Publications for the patient include *Help is On the Way* and *Who Am I?* (A medical emergency ID card is also available.) For the public, the booklet *What Is Myasthenia Gravis?* is available, along with government publications on the subject. The film, "Strength for Tomorrow," is free to groups and for TV showings. Materials for professionals include a manual on diagnosis and management for the physician, a manual introducing the disease to nurses, a film on diagnosis and management, and reprints of professional journal articles and proceedings of Foundation symposia. Bibliographies for the professional are also available.

National Alliance for the Mentally
Ill (NAMI)
500 North Broadway
St. Louis, MO 63102
(314) 231-8600

Handicapping Conditions Served: Mental illness.

The Organization: The National Alliance for the Mentally Ill (NAMI) was created at a conference of independent self-help organizations held in September 1979. NAMI was formed to act as a collective voice for reforms in legislation, health care, and employment opportunities for the chronically mentally ill patient. NAMI's first priorities are to gain funding, to establish state chapters, and to formulate by-laws and establish classes of membership. Long range plans include: coordinating the activities of state and local advocacy groups; serving as an information clearinghouse on mental illness; and promoting legislation, quality institutional and noninstitutional care, research, and public education programs.

Information Services: Membership applications are available from NAMI. The organization publishes a newsletter twice yearly.

National ALS Foundation, Inc.
185 Madison Avenue
New York, NY 10016
(212) 679-4016

Handicapping Conditions Served: Amyotrophic lateral sclerosis (ALS).

The Organization: The Foundation was established in 1971 to help ALS families live with the disease, to educate the public about the nature of ALS, and to foster medical research on its cause and cure. In 1978 the Foundation instituted outpatient services in the neurological clinic at Mount Sinai Medical Center, New York City, where diagnosis and follow-up care are provided without cost to patients from anywhere in the United States. The Foundation continues to fund medical research, and is currently sponsoring a computerized study of ALS patients. Ten chapters offer counseling and referrals to medical facilities. The Foundation also has equipment—ranging from page turners to wheelchairs—for free loan, as available, to patients.

Information Services: Publications include *Home Care for the Patient with Amyotrophic Lateral Sclerosis* as well as brochures describing the disease and the activities of the Foundation. A newsletter, *National Update*, reports on current experimental research and activities of the Foundation and its chapters. Lists and catalogs of home care agencies, transportation facilities, manufacturers of mechanical aids, local ALS chapters, and equipment available for loan can be requested. Data compiled from patient questionnaires on 700 cases in the computerized study of ALS can be obtained in abstract form by researchers or other interested persons. There is no charge for information or services.

National Amputation Foundation (NAF)
12-45 150th Street
Whitestone, NY 11357
(212) 767-0596

Handicapping Conditions Served: Amputation.

The Organization: The National Amputation Foundation (NAF) was established to help the amputee adjust to his handicap by encouraging integration into the general community. To this end, NAF offers: volunteer assistance to new amputees in hospitals; monthly social meetings focusing on topics of concern to the amputee, such as legal rights, benefits, and employment; and training in the use of prosthetics. NAF operates its own prosthetic center for the manufacture and repair of artificial limbs.

Information Services: NAF provides information on veterans' benefits and refers the amputee to possible sources of financial aid, legal assistance, and employment services. The Foundation has a reference library on amputation and materials are available for loan to any interested person. A monthly newsletter covers the highlights of NAF meetings.

**National Association for Hearing
  and Speech Action (NAHSA)**
6110 Executive Boulevard
Suite 1000
Rockville, MD 20852
(301) 897-8682 (Voice/TTY)

Handicapping Conditions Served: Speech, language and hearing impairments.

The Organization: The National Association for Hearing and Speech Action is a membership organization of individuals with speech, hearing and language disorders and their families. NAHSA is primarily concerned with advocating for the rights of the communicatively impaired and with public information

27

activities. Its most recent effort has been a campaign to alert the hearing impaired that closed captioning, which prints dialogue across the screen, will be available for selected programs on television.

Information Services: A Hearing and Speech HELPline (the above number may be called collect) has been set up to handle specific questions about communication problems and how to find professional assistance. The Association distributes organizational brochures and information on closed captioning free, upon request.

**National Association for Sickle Cell
    Disease, Inc. (NASCD)
3460 Wilshire Blvd.
Suite 1012
Los Angeles, CA 90010**

Handicapping Conditions Served: Sickle cell disease (including sickle cell anemia, hemoglobin C, and thalassemia) and sickle cell trait.

The Organization: The National Association for Sickle Cell Disease (NASCD) is an organization of 60 community sickle cell programs located throughout the U.S. and in the Bahamas. The national office has an extensive public and professional education program about sickle cell disease, its variants, and sickle cell trait. It advocates to prevent employment discrimination and to provide appropriate insurance coverage for persons with sickle cell trait.

NASCD provides technical assistance to its affillitates and to groups interested in setting up community sickle cell programs. Affiliates conduct a variety of services, depending on the particular needs of the communities they serve. Services may include: sickle cell screening, counseling to parents who possess the sickle cell trait and to patients with sickle cell disease, blood banks, tutoring, vocational rehabilitation, transportation services, babysitting, etc. The national office and its affiliates provide training to genetic counselors in how to counsel persons with sickle cell trait.

Information Services: NASCD's information is directed to lay persons, physicians and other professionals, and sickle cell program administrators and volunteers. Lay materials include fact sheets, audiovisuals, color prints and brochures about sickle cell trait and anemia, thalassemia and hemoglobin C. *A Home Study Kit for Families* includes printed materials, cassettes, games and other learning devices to help parents and other family members cope with the problems of the child or the family members may have. Professional materials include reprints of articles for pediatricians and genetic counselors, and a variety of manuals on the establishment of sickle cell programs, laboratory procedures for detection of the disease, and guidelines for legislation. NASCD's scientific advisory board contributes news on the latest research developments in sickle cell disease to the organization's newsletter, *Viewpoint*. Materials are available to all persons for minimal fees.

**National Association for the
    Deaf-Blind (NADB)
2703 Forest Oak Circle
Norman, OK 73071
(405) 360-2580**

Handicapping Conditions Served: Deaf-blindness.

The Organization: The National Association for the Deaf-Blind (NADB) was founded in 1975 by parents as an advocacy organization to further educational, rehabilitation, and employment opportunities for the deaf-blind. At the local level, through its 10 regional directors, NADB encourages the formation of local parent advocacy groups and advises them. Three experimental workshops: Making a Family Work;

Advocacy; and Responsibilities of a Parent, are designed for parents to train other parents in advocacy leadership in all regions of the country.

Information Services: A large print newsletter is distributed to Association members and is available, on a limited basis, to professionals. It covers relevant legislation, benefits, court cases, and state and local workshops. Requests for information in other areas which affect the deaf-blind are answered if time and staff limitations allow. Regional directors provide information on local education and vocational rehabilitation facilities, and possible sources of financial assistance.

**National Association for Visually
   Handicapped (NAVH)
305 East 24th Street, 17-C
New York, NY 10010
(212) 889-3141**

Handicapping Conditions Served: Partial vision, defined as visual acuity of 20/60 or less in the better eye with the best possible lens correction, but with some useable, residual vision.

The Organization: The National Association for Visually Handicapped (NAVH) provides information and referral and direct services. The latter include: 1) printing and distributing large print textbooks, educational testing material, and books for pleasure reading; 2) offering a free loan library of large print books; 3) serving as advocate for partially seeing individuals to Federal, state, and local government agencies; 4) offering youth group programs and adult discussion groups in New York and San Francisco, and a parent discussion group in San Francisco; 5) offering counsel and guidance to adults with partial vision and their families, to families of children with partial vision, and to all professionals and paraprofessionals who work with the partially seeing.

Information Services: NAVH acts as a clearinghouse of information for all services available to the partially seeing from Federal, state, and local government agencies and from private sources. NAVH publishes informational materials, not available elsewhere, concerning the problems encountered by the partially seeing. The organization publishes two newsletters in large print, one for children and one for adults. The national office provides information and referral services to any inquirer outside the State of California (a San Francisco office serves that State). Information on commercially available large print reading material and various optical aids is also disseminated. Most printed materials are free of charge, although a nominal contribution is requested for some items. A contribution is welcomed for all services.

**National Association of Councils
   of Stutterers (NACS)
c/o Speech and Hearing Clinic
The Catholic University of America
Washington, DC 20064
(202) 635-5556**

Handicapping Conditions Served: Stuttering.

The Organization: The National Association of Councils of Stutterers (NACS) was established to help form local stuttering councils nationwide. There are 10 local member councils in the U.S., self-help groups which offer stutterers opportunities to share their communication experiences and to learn successful techniques of control from each other.

Information Services: NACS provides materials and suggestions to any group of stutterers interested in starting a local council. It refers stutterers to local self-help groups and to local accredited therapy services. Films on stuttering self-help and prevention of stuttering in children are available on a loan or rental basis from Seven Oaks Productions, 8811 Colesville Road, #G106, Silver Spring, MD 20910. NACS publishes a quarterly journal covering local council news and information, recent research on stuttering, and new stuttering therapies. For information, contact Michael Hartford, Executive Secretary, at the above address.

National Association of Patients on
   Hemodialysis and Transplantation (NAPHT)
505 Northern Boulevard
Great Neck, NY 11021
(516) 482-2720

Handicapping Conditions Served: Kidney diseases.

The Organization: The National Association of Patients on Hemodialysis and Transplantation is primarily a patient organization with approximately 10,000 members and 30 local chapters. Its purposes are: to inform the public and the patient about kidney disease; to stimulate public awareness of the need for kidney donors; to act as a consumer advocacy group at the Federal and local levels; and to provide a source of moral support to the kidney patient. The chapters function as mutual support groups; activities vary among them, but often include educational meetings with professional speakers, self-help meetings, hospital visitations to new kidney patients, group outings, and community awareness programs. NAPHT is working with vocational rehabilitation specialists to develop specific programs for the kidney patient.

Information Services: The national office supplies information about kidney diseases, treatments and patient rights issues. Publications include free pamphlets, such as *Living with Renal Failure, Renal Failure and Diabetes,* and a salt-potassium counter. *Dialysis Worldwide for the Traveling Patient* is a regularly updated source of information about dialysis centers which accept transient patients; and *State Renal Programs* provides information about benefits available from state agencies. *NAPHT News* is a quarterly magazine which features exercise and diet suggestions, travel tips and reports on medical developments for the renal patient.

National Association of the Deaf (NAD)
814 Thayer Avenue
Silver Spring, MD 20910
(301) 587-1788 (Voice or TTY)

Handicapping Conditions Served: Deafness, hearing impairment, and deaf-blindness.

The Organization: The National Association of the Deaf (NAD) is a consumer oriented organization for professionals and lay persons. It recommends and promotes legislation on behalf of deaf people in areas of education, rehabilitation, legal rights for the provision of interpreters, hearing aid regulation, and captioned television. NAD's Communication Skills Program sponsors a university oriented training program to upgrade instructional skills of teachers of sign language, develops appropriate curriculum and instructional materials for teachers, and conducts a professional evaluation and certification program for instructors in various sign systems. NAD screens and evaluates general entertainment motion pictures, and recommends films to be captioned by the Conference of Executives of American Schools of the Deaf under contract with the Department of Health, Education, and Welfare.

Information Services: NAD has information on where to find programs and services for the deaf, including: schools, camps, interpreters, homes for the aged deaf, devices to assist deaf persons, hearing-ear dogs, and individual professional providers from medical specialists to speech therapists. NAD compiled statistical information about the deaf in a 1974 National Census of the Deaf. Information regarding legislation and legal rights of the deaf is also available. NAD's 47 state affiliates specialize in information about rehabilitation centers and counseling services. General information is provided free to any inquirer.

The organization offers a series of workshops (most held at its biennial conference, but some offered at local meetings nationwide) for professionals and lay persons on such topics as legal concerns of the deaf, orientation to deafness, leadership training for deaf persons, and need for and implementation of mental health services for the deaf. A wide variety of books, audiovisual materials, and merchandise (stationery, bumper stickers, etc.) relating to deafness and sign language is available from the NAD Publishing Division. NAD publishes three periodicals for general audiences: *The Deaf American*, a monthly magazine highlighting the achievements of deaf individuals; *The Broadcaster*, a monthly newspaper covering legislative and legal issues; and *The Interstate*, a bimonthly newsletter, for members only, focusing on state issues and news. A general information packet for hearing persons interested in deafness and a similar packet for medical professionals which contains an NAD booklet, *Medical Aspects of Deafness*, are available free from the organization. NAD has an extensive library of more than 15,000 books and other materials related to deafness. Any interested person may have access to the NAD collection.

National Ataxia Foundation
6681 Country Club Drive
Minneapolis, MN 55427
(612) 546-6220

Handicapping Conditions Served: Hereditary ataxia and related conditions.

The Organization: The Foundation was established in 1957 to serve patients, identify persons at risk, educate the public and the medical community, and stimulate research. Twenty chapters throughout the country offer genetic counseling and moral support to affected families, make referrals to medical and other direct service providers, and raise funds for research grants. Semiannual free clinics are offered in Minneapolis and elsewhere in the country where diagnosis and other informational services are available from professionals experienced in work with this neurological disorder.

Information Services: Free booklets, brochures, and fact sheets are available on hereditary ataxia, spastic paraplegia, Charcot-Marie-Tooth disease, hereditary tremor, and Friedreich's ataxia. Membership information, a quarterly newsletter, and special publications for physicians may also be requested.

National Committee/Arts for
the Handicapped (NCAH)
1701 K Street, N.W.
Suite 801
Washington, DC 20006
(202) 223-8007

Handicapping Conditions Served: All handicaps.

The Organization: Established in 1974, the National Committee/Arts for the Handicapped (NCAH) is an educational affiliate of the Kennedy Center for the Performing Arts. It disseminates information about curriculum and instruction in the arts for handicapped people; supports model arts programs for the handicapped; and publicizes the need for the benefit of expanded arts opportunities for handicapped people. NCAH sponsors "Very Special Arts Festivals" in 75 sites across the country which offer inservice training to teachers and administrators, offer workshops and performances by visiting artists, and provide opportunities for handicapped children to demonstrate or perform in the arts arena. Mainly through grants provided by HEW's Bureau of Education for the Handicapped, NCAH conducts research in the areas of model arts programs for the handicapped and in preparation of personnel.

Information Services: The Committee has compiled lists of national, state, and local organizations with art programs for the handicapped, model sites and other programs which the NCAH recognizes for excellence, and sources of financial assistance for establishing programs and conducting research projects. Materials about NCAH research and demonstration projects are available free. Other publications are available for a nominal charge and include reviews of special projects, curriculum ideas for parents and teachers, resource guides and bibliographies. Brochures emphasizing the importance of art, music, dance, and drama for the handicapped are also available. For additional information, contact Ralph Nappi, Division Director, Resources and Information.

National Congress of Organizations of the Physically Handicapped, Inc.
(National COPH, Inc.)
101 Lincoln Park Boulevard
Rockford, IL 61102
(815) 964-9883

Handicapping Conditions Served: All physical handicaps.

The Organization: The National Congress of Organizations of the Physically Handicapped, Inc. is an umbrella organization for about 50 local organizations or associations for the physically handicapped. It serves these organizations by advising them in their daily operations, by coordinating the joint activities of member organizations, and by representing the legislative objectives of member organizations at the national and state levels.

Information Services: National COPH, Inc. acts as a clearinghouse for publications of member and nonmember organizations. It publishes a quarterly newsletter with information on developments in rehabilitation and on state and local legislation affecting the physically handicapped. For information, contact: Lee Fredric Wiedenhoefer, Executive Director.

National Council on Alcoholism,
Inc. (NCA)
733 Third Avenue
New York, NY 10017
(212) 986-4433

Handicapping Conditions Served: Alcoholism.

The Organization: Defining alcoholism as a treatable disease, NCA works with 200 affiliates to educate professionals as well as the public in early identification and treatment. NCA components include the American Medical Society on Alcoholism and the Research Society on Alcoholism, both of which publish research findings, and the National Nurses' Society on Alcoholism. NCA works through its affiliates at local levels to develop programs for women; for labor and employer organizations in government, business, and industry; and for youth, minority and indigent populations.

Information Services: As an information clearinghouse on alcoholism, the Council maintains a library of journals, books, pamphlets, and government reports for on-site research. Specific inquiries, statistical data, and referrals to local facilities or resource persons are handled by the Library/Information Service by phone or letter. Prepared bibliographies, indexes, abstracts of scientific articles and fact sheets on education and prevention programs can be requested; a number of these materials are also available in Spanish. A monthly newsletter reports on research in the *Physician's Alcohol Newsletter,* and *Alcohol:*

Clinical and Experimental Research may be ordered by subscription or single copy. The NCA also publishes the *Labor-Management Journal* for employers and unions which participate in alcoholism control programs. A catalog of publications include titles of interest to clergy, courts, families, youth and women as well as pamphlets by Alcoholics Anonymous. There is a nominal charge for most booklets.

National Easter Seal Society
2023 West Ogden Avenue
Chicago, IL 60612
(312) 243-8400

Handicapping Conditions Served: All handicaps.

The Organization: The Society is the nation's largest and oldest (1919) voluntary health agency providing direct rehabilitation services to persons with disabilities. Some 1,124 member groups, organized on a state and local basis, provide over 2,000 programs which include comprehensive medical or vocational rehabilitation facilities, recreation, housing, transportation, equipment loans, public education, advocacy and other services for the prevention and treatment of disabling conditions.

The National Society, acting as headquarters for the federation of local and state organizations, conducts national public awareness and fund raising campaigns, disseminates information, and through its Research Foundation, awards grants for research into the causes, treatment, and rehabilitation of disabling conditions.

Information Services: An interdisciplinary journal, *Rehabilitation Literature,* which has been published for the past 40 years, contains original articles, book reviews, and abstracts of current professional literature. The Center has compiled bibliographies from the entries in the journal in subject areas of interest to rehabilitation personnel, persons with disabilities and their families, and Easter Seal staff and volunteers. The National Easter Seal Society publishes a variety of books, pamphlets and reprints for professionals, parents and persons with disabilities. Its catalog lists publications related to: 1) advocacy, 2) attitudes, 3) barrier-free environment, 4) dental care, 5) disabling conditions, 6) education, 7) independent living, 8) prevention, 9) recreation and camping, 10) sexual adjustment, 11) social and psychological aspects, and 12) volunteers.

For additional information about publications, contact the Program Services Department.

National Federation of the Blind (NFB)
1800 Johnson Street
Baltimore, MD 21230
(301) 659-9314

Handicapping Conditions Served: Blindness.

The Organization: The National Federation of the Blind (NFB) is a membership organization with 51 state and 400 local chapters. NFB keeps up with Federal and state legislation affecting the blind and state services for the blind. It acts as a legislative resource for its chapters and represents the needs of blind people through advocacy and representation in discrimination cases. It attempts to arouse public awareness of the potential and accomplishments of the blind through public service messages. State and local chapters are active in developing local projects to improve conditions for the blind in areas such as mass transit, employment, and library services. Members contact newly blinded persons to help them with problems of adjustment.

Information Services: NFB conducts seminars on services available to the blind and what the law provides for in each state. Its **National Blindness Information Center** will attempt to answer any questions about blindness and the rights of the blind by phone or mail. More than 50 publications are available from NFB; some are free. NFB publishes a monthly magazine, *The Braille Monitor* (available in print, disc, and braille), which reports on problems, progress, activities, and new technologies related to blindness. State and local chapters refer inquirers to appropriate direct service providers.

**National Foundation for Jewish Genetic
    Diseases (NFJGD)**
609 Fifth Avenue
Suite 1200
New York, NY 10017
(212) 753-5155

Handicapping Conditions Served: Jewish genetic diseases.

The Organization: The National Foundation for Jewish Genetic Diseases (NFJGD) was established to raise funds for and inform the public about genetic diseases which afflict Ashkenazi Jews (descendants of Jews from Eastern and Central Europe). These diseases have been identified as familial dysautonomia, torsion dystonia, Gaucher's disease, Bloom's diseas, Niemann-Pick disease, Tay Sachs and Mucolipidosis IV.

Information Services: The Foundation provides fact sheets, reprints, and audiovisual materials about Jewish genetic diseases upon request. Materials describe the diseases and recommend genetic counseling to prospective parents. A semiannual newsletter covers activities of the Foundation. NFJGD sponsors symposia and has a speakers' bureau available to present programs on the diseases and their effects. NFJGD refers parents of afflicted children to medical specialists.

NFJGD has sponsored the writing of two books, *Genetic Disorders Among the Jewish People* (Johns Hopkins University Press), and *Genetic Diseases Affecting Ashkenazi Jews* (Raven Press); these are available available from the publishers.

**National Fraternal Society
    of the Deaf (NFSD)**
1300 W. Northwest Highway
Mt. Prospect, IL 60056
(312) 392-9282 (Voice)
(312) 392-1409 (TTY)

Handicapping Conditions Served: Deafness and hearing impairments.

The Organization: Organized and administered by deaf people, the organization was originally founded to provide life insurance coverage for deaf people who were not eligible to buy from established companies. Membership, which entails purchase of insurance, is open to all hearing impaired persons, their relatives and others involved in the field of deafness—between the ages of 0 and 60. NFSD advocates the rights of deaf people to drive and obtain auto insurance and works to eliminate discrimination in employment, education, and legal proceedings. The organization also awards scholastic and athletic achievement, and sponsors local and national social activities.

Information Services: A field force of trained representatives exists to offer detailed information and explanation of a variety of insurance investments and estate planning to deaf and hearing impaired persons. Consumer education is also conducted through local chapters and through the bimonthly magazine, *The Frat*, which carries news of the Society's insurance, social, and advocacy activities. The national office maintains an extensive library collection of monographs and pamphlets relating to deafness, which is available to any person or group for reference or research.

National Genetics Foundation, Inc.
9 West 57th Street
New York, NY 10019
(212) 759-4432

Handicapping Conditions Served: All genetic disorders.

The Organization: The Foundation was incorporated in 1953 as a nonprofit, voluntary clearinghouse of information and referrals on the more than 2,000 genetic disorders which affect an estimated five percent of the population. The Foundation sponsors a Network of Genetic Counseling Treatment Centers at 60 medical centers throughout the country where diagnostic tests and genetic counseling are available to parents and prospective parents at risk for genetic disorders. The Foundation offers preliminary counseling and assembles a family medical history which is then forwarded to the patient's nearest diagnostic and treatment center. Even though that center may not specialize in the particular disorder, the patient's physician may avail himself of the expertise of scientists working on the disease through the exchanges of blood and tissue samples with other medical centers in the Network. Counseling is offered at the local center on the basis of information available through the Network. While there is usually a charge for laboratory work and direct services of local centers, the Foundation's information and referral services are free. The Foundation also conducts education programs for physicians as well as the general public on legal, ethical, and other questions relating to medical genetics.

Information Services: Direct inquiries from patients or physicians are handled by professional staff of the Foundation. Brochures are available including: *How Genetic Disease Can Affect You and Your Family; Can Genetic Counseling Help You?; Genetic Counseling and Treatment Network; For the Concerned Couple Planning a Family;* and *Should You Consider Amniocentesis?*

National Hemophilia Foundation (NHF)
25 West 39th Street
New York, NY 10018
(212) 869-9740

Handicapping Conditions Served: Hemophilia.

The Organization: The objective of the National Hemophilia Foundation (NHF) and its 50 chapters is to improve and expand medical treatment and supportive services to the hemophiliac. HNF also sponsors research in the prevention and treatment of hemophilia. Chapters provide varying direct services. Some are comprehensive care treatment centers; some are affiliated with treatment centers. Most chapters sponsor scholarships and "camperships" to hemophiliac youths.

Information Services: The **NHF Clearinghouse** is a newly established information center of the Foundation, funded by the Department of Health, Education, and Welfare. An annotated compilation of 30 NHF publications and 4 NHF audiovisuals, together with an order form, is available from the Clearinghouse. Publications include general information on hemophilia for patients and their families, such as sources of possible financial assistance, and a variety of technical literature on care and treatment. Some professional materials are devoted to specialty areas such as dentistry, orthopedics, surgery, and physical therapy. NHF also publishes study reports, conference proceedings, bibliographies, and service directories (notably *Guide for Traveling Hemophiliacs, State and Federal Resources Guide for Hemophiliacs,* and *Directory of Hemophilia Treatment Centers*). The Clearinghouse has compiled a cumulative list of health educational materials related to hemophilia, published by pharmaceutical companies, blood banking organizations, and government agencies.

NHF chapters refer hemophiliacs and their families to appropriate direct care facilities and to possible sources of financial assistance.

**National Huntington's Disease
  Association**
128A East 74th Street
New York, NY 10021
(212) 966-4320

Handicapping Conditions Served: Huntington's Disease (HD).

The Organization: Organized in 1976 by families, professionals, and citizens concerned with HD, the Association now has 11 chapters and 20 area representatives. The Association offers postdoctoral fellowships in HD and related disorders. Members offer patients moral support, and referrals to local facilities and to genetic counselors who assist the patient's family to identify the risks to themselves and future generations. Public awareness is another important activity of the Association, which works to remove the stigma that has for centuries surrounded victims who often exhibit symptoms of chorea ("dance" like muscular spasms) and pronounced personality change. The Association also supports medical research by fund raising and collection of autopsy brain tissue for scientists who are working on HD.

Information Services: Information brochures explaining the inheritance and effects of the disease, a manual for medical professionals, a booklet on clinical care (for physicians), reprints of articles about HD and the Association, and a list of local chapters and representatives are available on request, along with membership information and a quarterly newsletter. Referrals can also be made to local medical and nursing home facilities.

National Kidney Foundation (NKF)
2 Park Avenue
New York, NY 10016
(212) 889-2210

Handicapping Conditions Served: Genitourinary disorders.

The Organization: Since 1950 the Foundation has supported a variety of programs in treatment, research, and education of both the public and professionals. The Organ Donor Program works through 53 affiliates to gather kidneys and other organs for transplant. Support of blood banks for dialysis patients, administration of detection and screening programs, and staffing of information and referral offices along with advocacy and public information activities are among the activities of Foundation affiliates. NKF sponsors symposia, conferences, and meetings for medical and allied health professionals. Education of professionals is provided by five Councils of the Foundation: Dialysis and Transplantation, Nephrology Social Workers, Renal Nutrition, Urology, and Nephrology Nurses and Technicians.

Information Services: Affiliates provide counseling and referrals to local resources for patients and their families. Publications include *The Kidney*, a bimonthly scientific report on research and clinical developments in all aspects of kidney disease, and *Perspectives*, a journal featuring information on legislation and advances in social work and practice as they relate to patients. Information brochures for patients and their families include (among others): *What Everyone Should Know about Kidneys, Childhood Nephrosis*, and *High Blood Pressure and Your Kidneys*. A newsletter reports on news of affiliates' activities.

National Multiple Sclerosis Society
205 East 42nd Street
New York, NY 10017
(212) 986-3240

Handicapping Conditions Served: Multiple sclerosis and related diseases.

The Organization: Funding of research, public and professional education, the design of rehabilitative and psychosocial programs and advocacy are activities of the Society, which also offers other direct services to patients through 150 local chapters and branches. A Washington office is active in advocacy of federal legislation affecting MS persons. Among the programs offered by chapters are a variety of counseling and referral services; many offer group aquatics and other social/recreational support, and MS home care courses for families and friends of patients developed in cooperation with the American National Red Cross. Seventy-five clinical treatment centers are supported by local chapters in 30 states.

Information Services: Publications for the general public include such titles as *What Everyone Should Know about Multiple Sclerosis* and *Living With MS: A Practical Guide*. Patient information includes home exercise manuals for ambulatory and nonambulatory persons, pamphlets on mental and emotional health, nutrition, careers for the homebound, newsletters and information on current research. Professionals may request publications on treatment, nursing care, and group counseling, as well as reprints of journal articles. Referrals, information on technical aids and equipment, and order lists for free publications can be obtained at chapters as well as from the national office.

National Neurofibromatosis
Foundation (NNFF)
340 East 80th Street, #21-H
New York, NY 10021

Handicapping Conditions Served: Neurofibromatosis (Von Recklinghausen's Disease).

The Organization: Neurofibromatosis (NF) is an inherited neurological disorder which can affect all areas of the nervous system and the skin. Symptoms of the disorder usually begin in childhood or adolescence when multiple benign tumors appear on the brain, spinal cord and skin; the nerves controlling vision and hearing are often affected. The Foundation was established in 1978 to provide information to patients and their families, physicians, and other professionals and to promote and support scientific research on the cause, prevention and treatment of NF. Thus far, the Foundation's activities include public awareness campaigns, professional workshops on NF (jointly sponsored by the National Cancer Institute), and an epidemiological survey of patients with the disorder—the data to be utilized for future research. NNFF soon expects to be able to provide research funds as seed grants to institutions. NNFF members include patients, physicians and social service agencies.

Information Services: NNFF publishes a fact sheet on NF and an organizational newsletter which includes information about patient rights and physicians responses to patient inquiries about NF, and collects professional literature related to NF and makes copies available to physicians and health workers. The Foundation assists patients in finding medical, social and genetic counseling.

National Parkinson Foundation
1501 N.W. Ninth Avenue
Miami, FL 33136
(305) 547-6666

Handicapping Conditions Served: Parkinson's disease, multiple sclerosis, and related neurological disorders.

The Organization: The National Parkinson Foundation supports the National Parkinson Institute, which provides outpatient diagnostic, treatment, and rehabilitation services to patients with Parkinson's disease and related neurological diseases, such as multiple sclerosis. The Foundation also funds the Bob Hope Parkinson Research Center, which investigates the causes and treatment of Parkinson's disease. The

Center has recently become affiliated with the University of Miami Department of Neurology, which will conduct research into other neurological disorders as well. The Foundation offers research grants to other medical centers in the area of Parkinson's disease.

Information Services: The Foundation publishes a periodic research newsletter, of interest to both lay and professional readers. Additional publications include *What the Patient Should Know about Parkinson's Disease* and *Psychological Factors in the Management of Parkinson's Disease*. All Foundation publications are free in limited quantities.

National Retinitis Pigmentosa
Foundation (RP Foundation)
Rolling Park Building
8331 Mindale Circle
Baltimore, MD 21207

Handicapping Conditions Served: Blindness and visual impairments, caused by inherited retinal degenerative diseases.

The Organization: The National Retinitis Pigmentosa Foundation funds research in retinitis pigmentosa (RP) and other retinal degenerative diseases. It funds eight research centers in the U.S. and England—each involved in different but coordinated areas of investigation into retinal degenerative diseases. The RP Foundation maintains a national confidential registry of RP affected persons for statistical and eventual use in its clinical research. In addition the Foundation has initiated an RP Retina Donor Program to assist the researchers' efforts. The Organization's 42 chapters are involved in a variety of activities including information and referral, experience sharing, and fund raising. Furthermore, the National RP Foundation is a part of the International Retinitis Pigmentosa Association—a coalition of countries which coordinate research on a worldwide basis.

Information Services: Twenty-two Volunteer Information Resource Centers (VIRC) plus the 42 chapters provide referral service to rehabilitation, psychological, medical and vocational counseling agencies. The RP Foundation publishes several information fact sheets, an annual report and a quarterly newsletter for the lay reader. The RP Foundation holds regional educational workshops for volunteers and professionals, where leading speakers in the field of RP are featured.

National Society for Autistic
Children (NSAC)
1234 Massachusetts Avenue, N.W.
Suite 1017
Washington, DC 20005
(202) 783-0125

Handicapping Conditions Served: Autism.

The Organization: The National Society for Autistic Children (NSAC) is an organization of parents, professionals, and other interested people who work for legislation, education, and research for the benefit of all children with severe behavior disorders. Advocacy on the national, state, and local levels, particularly in the area of education, is a primary function of the organization. NSAC sponsors a job exchange, matching qualified professionals with available openings. The 57 local chapters of NSAC support various direct services, such as recreational programs and group homes (residences for 8 to 12 children).

Information Services: The organization publishes general information pamphlets defining autism and suggesting management techniques. NSAC's **Information and Referral Service**, located at the above address, has specific information available, including: 1) names, addresses, and other information about day and residential programs and camps which admit children with autism; 2) cities and states where autistic children are educated in public schools; 3) a list of facilities which admit autistic adolescents and adults; 4) how to effectively organize to get community services for children with autism; 5) legislative information at national and state levels; 6) suggestions for sources of funds, public and private; 7) a list of colleges and universities which offer training in the field of autism; 8) income tax information for parents; and 9) a list of contacts and societies for children with autism in other countries. The service also keeps an informal list of research projects being conducted in the area of autism.

NSAC publishes three newsletters: one, an advocacy publication for lay readers; one for teachers of autistic children; and one intended for local chapters and other organizations involved in problems of the autistic child. A wide variety of books about autism for the professional and lay reader are selected and distributed by NSAC's bookstore. Copies of professional papers delivered at the organization's annual meetings are also available from the bookstore.

**National Society to Prevent
    Blindness (NSPB)
79 Madison Avenue
New York, NY 10016
(212) 684-3505**

Handicapping Conditions Served: Prevention of blindness and visual impairments.

The Organization: This organization works to prevent blindness by sponsoring community screening and testing programs, public and professional education, and research. Community programs, carried out through 25 affiliated volunteer state agencies, concentrate on health education and free screening for the public. These programs aim to detect, control, correct, or prevent glaucoma and cataract blindness; eye problems in children; eye accidents; and blindness caused by hereditary and congenital conditions, diabetes, and muscular degeneration. NSPB works for the implementation of laws for eye protection in hazardous environments. It funds research in eye care and disease prevention.

Information Services: NSPB provides answers to specific questions about eye diseases, eye safety, vision defects, and eye checkups when queried by mail. It publishes brochures and pamphlets on various subjects, such as glaucoma, cataracts, sunglasses, and TV and your eyes, providing single copies of most materials at no charge. Also free are reprints on intraocular lenses and diabetic retinopathy, a home eye exam for parents to test children, and low-cost curriculum aids for teachers. A complete catalog of NSPB publications and films is available.

**National Spinal Cord Injury
    Foundation
369 Elliot Street
Newton Upper Falls, MA 02164
(617) 964-0521**

The Handicapping Conditions Served: Spinal cord injuries caused by trauma and disease.

The Organization: Founded by the Paralyzed Veterans of America in 1948, the National Paraplegia Foundation in 1979 merged with the New England Spinal Cord Injury Foundation and adopted the present name. Dedicated to "care, cure, and coping," the Foundation works through its 67 chapters to develop comprehensive systems of quality care for paraplegics and quadriplegics. Care is offered as a direct service by some chapters which give individual case consultations and advise on case management of the newly injured. Other chapters make referrals to direct service providers. All chapters emphasize personal contact between persons with spinal cord injuries and involve them in all aspects of Foundation activities. **Cure** is the goal of the research division which offers fellowships to neuroscientists who are working in the field of repair or regeneration of the spinal cord. Regional seminars and an annual conference give professionals, constituents, and other interested persons an opportunity to exchange and compare new developments in technological, environmental, and medical research. The Foundation functions as a clearinghouse of information for medical and other health care workers. **Coping** with the disability is facilitated by peer counseling; public awareness; and environmental barrier removal. Some chapters sponsor independent living rehabilitation programs and more of these are being developed for the severely physically disabled (quadriparetic).

Information Services: Information on independent living rehabilitation programs, self-help devices, equipment, transportation, employment, education, personal care, and referrals is available from the national office and through chapters. Individual case consultations and case management advice can also be requested; contacts can be arranged for person to person assistance and peer counseling, if appropriate. Publications include *Cost Effectiveness of Spinal Cord Injury Center Treatment; Paraplegia Life,* a bimonthly magazine; regional and national resource directories, and handbooks on nursing, personal care, and nutrition. Interested persons may also request bibliographies of current and relevant research.

National Stuttering Project (NSP)
656A 8th Avenue
San Francisco, CA 94118
(415) 387-7065

Handicapping Conditions Served: Stuttering.

The Organization: Established in 1977, NSP is a self-help group which offers a program of self therapy for stuttering in conjunction with the Speech Foundation of America. Local chapter meetings, special programs, and workshops provide opportunities for stutterers to express themselves and work through the problem in a supportive environment. NSP offers consultations in program development and technical assistance to school districts, speech clinics, hospitals, rehabilitation centers, and other agencies involved in speech services. Committed to consumer advocacy, NSP gathers and disseminates information about the professional community and advises members on how to be wise consumers of speech and related therapies. Status as members at large, a newsletter, and a person to person correspondents' program serve interested persons who are not affiliated with local chapters.

Information Services: Publications include pamphlets and article reprints with such titles as: *Shopping for a Speech Pathologist, Suggestions for Parents,* and *A Personal Journey through Stuttering.* A tape series and the handbook, *Self Therapy for Stuttering,* are available at nominal cost. NSP has a Speech Pathology Referral Service which provides information on experienced speech therapists. Speakers and slide show presentations may be requested by schools and other organizations.

National Tay-Sachs and Allied Diseases
   Association, Inc.
122 East 42nd Street
New York, NY 10017
(212) 661-2780

Handicapping Conditions Served: Tay-Sachs and other inborn errors of metabolism.

The Organization: Founded in 1957 as a parents' group to encourage medical research on Tay-Sachs disease, the Association has expanded its concerns to public and professional education about the disease and its detection and to the assurance of quality control of screening facilities. Screening for possible carriers of the Tay-Sachs gene and genetic counseling services are offered throughout the country.

Information Services: Brochures for lay and professional persons describe the disease and recommend preventive measures. A list of Tay-Sachs screening centers in the U.S. and Canada is also available. Professional papers and bibliographies on Tay-Sachs may be obtained from the Association at a minimal charge.

New parents of Tay-Sachs children are referred to a member of the Association's "peer group" for support and advice on management and appropriate medical channels to pursue.

**National Tuberous Sclerosis
    Association, Inc. (NTSA)**
P.O. Box 159
Laguna Beach, CA 92652
(714) 494-8900

Handicapping Conditions Served: Tuberous sclerosis (TS).

The Organization: The Association was founded in 1975 by parents and concerned physicians of patients with this genetic disorder which results in tumors or malformations in the nervous system and skin, convulsions, skin lesions, and—in severe cases—mental retardation. Accurate diagnosis, anticonvulsant therapy, and early developmental intervention are the goals of the organization. Dissemination of information to the medical profession as well as to parents and the general public, advancement of research by fund raising, and annual meetings for researchers and for the Association's membership of parents and professionals implement these goals. The Association has established a national Human Neurospecimen Bank and a case registry to assist scientists in their research. The members of the Association offer counseling, referral, and support services to other families of TS patients.

Information Services: Brochures and pamphlets for parents, reprints of articles on clinical research for physicians, and fact sheets describing symptoms and genetics of TS are available; request the publications list for titles. The Association publishes a quarterly newsletter and maintains a speakers bureau.

The Orton Society (OS)
8415 Bellona Lane
Towson, MD 21204
(301) 296-0232

Handicapping Conditions Served: Dyslexia.

The Organization: The Orton Society (OS) is an international membership organization for professionals and parents of dyslexic children. Its purposes are to disseminate information related to dyslexia, and to assist reading disabled children and adults in finding facilities for diagnosis, remediation, and tutoring. OS has 27 volunteer branches which serve the needs of their individual communities by offering guidance, workshops, and seminars.

Information Services: OS can provide some general information to inquirers by phone or by letter; most information requests are met through a variety of OS publications on dyslexia and related learning disabilities. The *OS Bulletin* is a compilation of scientific papers delivered at its annual conference, containing therapy applications and articles about the state of the art. Audiotapes of individual conference papers are available.

**Osteogenesis Imperfecta Foundation,
    Inc.**
632 Center Street
Van Wert, OH 45891
(419) 238-0993

Handicapping Conditions Served: Osteogenesis Imperfecta (brittle bones disease).

The Organization: The Foundation was organized in 1970 by parents of children suffering from this genetic defect. Characterized by fragility of bone and often by stunted growth, the condition displays a wide range of severity. Management of the disease and treatment of symptoms, which may include hearing and dental problems as well as frequent fractures, is now available at many hospitals and medical centers. Genetic counseling is another service offered to affected families. Information about these medical facilities and services, care and management techniques, and equipment is available from the Foundation office or any of the 12 local chapters. Public awareness and fund raising to support research are other activities of the organization. Members are adult patients as well as parents of children with the disease.

Information Services: Pamphlets describing the disease and its management; reprints of articles by parents, researchers, and health care professionals; a quarterly newsletter, *Breakthrough*; and referrals to local chapters and medical facilities are available from the Foundation president, Mrs. Gemma Geisman, at the above address.

Paralyzed Veterans of America (PVA)
4350 East West Highway
Suite 900
Washington, DC 20014
(301) 652-2135

Handicapping Conditions Served: Paralysis.

The Organization: Paralyzed Veterans of America (PVA) is a national service organization for paralyzed veterans with offices in each of the Veterans Administration's (VA) 18 Spinal Cord Injury Centers and in 30 VA regional offices and outpatient clinics. PVA operates as an information and advocacy agency, and supports and funds research in treatment, rehabilitation, and regeneration of spinal cord injury. A national advocacy program focuses on transportation, architectural barriers, wheelchair design, and employment and educational opportunities. PVA representatives plead claims for paralyzed veterans before government agencies. The organization has 34 local chapters in the U.S. that help the PVA carry out its programs. One of PVA's chapter oriented programs trains nurses in the care and treatment of spinal cord injury patients. PVA sponsors and supports wheelchair sports and recreation.

Information Services: PVA National Service Officers meet with the paralyzed veteran, assess his needs, and offer assistance and advice on legal benefits, rehabilitation, medication, and supplies available to him through the VA. If not eligible for VA benefits, the paralyzed veteran will be referred to other sources of possible assistance. Some local PVA chapters offer similar services.

PVA publishes a monthly magazine of information and entertainment and several pamphlets, including *An Introduction to Paraplegia, Wheelchair in a Home,* and *Highway Rest Areas for Handicapped Travelers.*

Parkinson's Disease Foundation, Inc.
William Black Medical Research Building
Columbia University Medical Center
640 W. 168th Street
New York, NY 10032
(212) 923-4700

Handicapping Conditions Served: Parkinson's disease.

The Organization: The Parkinson's Disease Foundation is primarily a research organization. It supports the Parkinson Research Laboratories at Columbia University Medical Center, where research is conducted in neuropharmacology, neurophysiology, neuropathology, and neurovirology. In 1960, the Foundation established a Brain Bank at Columbia University Medical School to give scientists the opportunity to study the brains of deceased Parkinson patients. The Foundation awards research grants and fellowships to investigators at Columbia and other medical schools. It sponsors symposia where scientists from the United States, Europe, and the Orient present findings of their long-term studies of Parkinson's disease.

Information Services: Proceedings from the symposia and other reports are published and distributed to all medical practitioners and institutions requesting them. For the lay and professional inquirer, the Foundation provides general information about Parkinson's disease. Three booklets are published by the Foundation specifically for the patient and his family: *The Parkinson Patient at Home; Exercises for the Parkinson Patient;* and *Parkinson's Disease: Progress, Promise and Hope.* A film is available on loan to health care groups and groups of patients, "Management of Parkinson's Disease and Syndrome with Levadopa." For information, contact Mrs. Dinah T. Orr, Executive Director.

People First International, Inc.
P.O. Box 12642
Salem, OR 97309
(503) 378-5143

Handicapping Conditions Served: Mental retardation and developmental disabilities.

The Organization: People First International is an organization of mentally retarded and developmentally disabled individuals who meet to learn leadership skills and how to advocate for themselves. People First began in Salem, Oregon, in 1973. Since then, more than 50 local chapters have been set up across the U.S. and in Canada. The national office provides assistance through consultation and workshops to groups wishing to establish chapters.

Information Services: Information about People First and how to set up programs is available from the organization. Materials include a "how-to" booklet, an officer's booklet, and a leisure time brochure, a film and several articles about the organization.

Prader-Willi Syndrome Association
5515 Malibu Drive
Edina, MN 55436
(612) 933-0113

Handicapping Conditions Served: Prader-Willi syndrome.

The Organization: Prader-Willi syndrome is a very rare condition which results from a birth defect. Those with this sporadically occurring disorder suffer obesity, short stature, poor muscle tone, and mental retardation. Association members are parents and professionals, who share knowledge and experience about the syndrome and how to manage it. Parent groups across the country hold informal meetings and often invite professional speakers to address them.

Information Services: The Association's newsletter contains tips from parents and professionals on management of a Prader-Willi syndrome child; diet is emphasized. *Prader-Willi Syndrome: A Handbook for Parents* contains information on behavior and learning capacity of the Prader-Willi child as well as tips on management, diet and exercise. The Handbook is available through the Association's newsletter, *The Gathered View*, 26931 S.E. 403rd, Enumclaw, WA 98022, for $2.00 for members and $3.50 for nonmembers.

The Association provides information to parents regarding physicians or hospitals with specific knowledge of the syndrome.

**Recovery, Inc., The Association of Nervous
and Former Mental Patients
116 South Michigan Avenue
Chicago, IL 60603
(312) 263-2292**

Handicapping Conditions Served: Emotional illness.

The Organization: Founded in 1937 to provide self help after care for released patients of psychiatrist Abraham Low, the organization uses Low's techniques of describing and coping with daily problems to prevent relapse or chronicity. All leadership is voluntary and groups follow procedures established by Dr. Low. Health care professionals are welcome as observers, but weekly meetings are conducted by members who are lay leaders and former patients. It is not necessary to have been under the treatment of a physician or to have been hospitalized to join Recovery; many members come through personal referrals or publicity as well as professional referral. There are 1,000 chapters in the U.S., Canada, Ireland, the United Kingdom, and Puerto Rico.

Information Services: The techniques on which the organization is based are presented in the handbook by Dr. Low, *Mental Health through Will Training* (available also in Spanish and French). Other Low lectures are available on cassettes or records; topics range from "The Fear of Life Ebbing Away" to "The Obsession of Being Contaminated." Pamphlets on the organization, a bimonthly newsletter, reprints of articles describing the organization, a publications list, and a directory of group meetings can be requested. The organization prefers to offer demonstration meetings instead of speakers at gatherings of professionals or for other interested organizations. Contact the headquarters office for information on this service.

**Rehabilitation International USA (RIUSA)
20 West 40th Street
New York, NY 10018
(212) 869-9907**

Handicapping Conditions Served: All handicaps.

The Organization: Rehabilitation International USA (RIUSA) is the U.S. representative of Rehabilitation International (RI), which has more than 60 member countries. RIUSA provides a link between the U.S. rehabilitation community (including the disabled and professional organizations and facilities which serve the disabled) and rehabilitation developments and services in other countries. One of RISUA's major concerns is in the area of travel and, through its **Access to the Skies Program**, it is cooperating with the aircraft industry in trying to standardize designs to make commercial aircraft accessible for disabled persons.

Information Services: RIUSA refers the disabled person and rehabilitation professional to contacts in other countries who are knowledgeable about specific services and opportunities for the disabled, such as educational and treatment facilities. It provides information about the process of finding a job in the rehabilitation field overseas. The organization collects information on independent living programs and on employment conditions for disabled people abroad.

RIUSA has a film rental library which houses 150 films on such subjects as rehabilitation training programs for professionals, physical therapy techniques, the use of prosthetics, and overcoming architectural barriers. A *REHABFILM Newsletter* covers audiovisual materials in the rehabilitation field.

RIUSA publishes *REHABILITATION/WORLD*, a quarterly professional journal which reports on innovative rehabilitation techniques, programs and devices in other countries. Annual directories published in the journal include: "The International Directory of Access Guides," a listing of more than 325 cities around the world which publish access guides for the elderly and the handicapped; and a "Directory of U.S. Rehabilitation Facilities Which Welcome Foreign and American Professional Visitors." RIUSA also distributes the *International Rehabilitation Review*, published by Rehabilitation International, to its members throughout the United States.

Sensory Aids Foundation (SAF)
399 Sherman Ave., Suite 12
Palo Alto, CA 94306
(415) 329-0430

Handicapping Conditions Served: Blindness and visual impairments.

The Organization: The Sensory Aids Foundation (SAF) is a nonprofit organization in operation since 1972, which introduces employers to the kinds of services and equipment they need in order to employ blind persons. Major services provided are: (1) employer orientation to sensory aids equipment used in making jobs accessible for blind and visually impaired persons; (2) identification of specific jobs which blind and visually impaired persons may perform competitively; and (3) identification of equipment used by blind and visually impaired persons. Other undertakings of SAF are sensitivity sessions on the employment of the blind for employers, and conferences on new sensory aids equipment produced by manufacturers in the U.S.A.

Information Services: Services are provided to potential employers, rehabilitation counselors, and anyone interested in working with visually handicapped persons. SAF publishes the *Sensory Aids Foundation Report* which includes information on the Foundation's current activities. New equipment is listed in their *Sensory Aids for Employment of Blind and Visually Impaired Persons: A Resource Guide*, with descriptions of 130 devices produced by U.S. manufacturers.

Society for the Rehabilitation
   of the Facially Disfigured
550 First Avenue
New York, NY 10016
(212) 679-1534

Handicapping Conditions Served: Facial disfigurement and deformities of the hand and upper extremities.

The Organization: The Society was founded to establish new treatment facilities and to encourage training in reconstructive plastic surgery as a means of aiding victims of facial disfigurement. The Society's Institute of Reconstructive Plastic Surgery at New York University Medical Center functions as a center for clinical services, professional training, and medical research, in association with several associated plastic surgery clinics in the New York metropolitan area. Research emphasizes three major areas: tissue and organ transplantation, microsurgery, and replantation of amputated fingers, hands, and other parts. A formal residency training program, approved by the AMA, is also offered. Special rehabilitation programs are available for those with congenital defects and cleft palate, and for hand, eye, and cancer surgery patients. Speech rehabilitation is emphasized, and the services of mental health professionals and vocational consultants are offered to assist with vocational problems.

Information Services: The Society routinely refers those interested in direct services to local plastic surgeons and clinics. Assistance is provided, if needed, in locating help to pay for the rehabilitation. Individual case reviews and recommendations are sometimes made by teams of specialists from the Institute. If the case is of such a serious nature that only the Institute could help, families are advised of the cost. Fact sheets describing the services of the Institute are available, as well as brochures and pamphlets describing the range of possibilities of such surgery, and giving selected patient histories from the Institute's files. A bibliography of publications by Institute physicians is also available.

Spina Bifida Association of America (SBAA)
343 South Dearborn Street
Suite 319
Chicago, IL 60604
(312) 663-1562

Handicapping Conditions Served: Spina bifida.

The Organization: Organized in 1974 as an outgrowth of the National Easter Seal Society, the SBAA began and continues a primary emphasi· on local parent and patient support groups. Activities also include public education, advocacy, and sponsorship of an annual conference for professionals and lay persons on medical, social, educational, and legal issues relating to this disability. A Medical Advisory Board identifies national medical needs and evaluates current medical advances, reporting on these to the membership. The Professional Advisory Board for Education studies current educational programs for children with spina bifida. SBAA continues to work closely with the National Easter Seal Society and the March of Dimes Birth Defects Foundation.

Information Services: Publications and public education media materials are available through 100 local chapters in the U.S. and Canada; chapters also sponsor parent, teenage, and young adult support groups. Publications include *The Child with Spina Bifida; By, For and With Young Adults with Spina Bifida;* a bimonthly newsletter, *The Pipeline;* and manuals for parents and teachers. Material on organizing SBAA chapters, copy for radio spots, publicity and media presentations, and a directory of chapters can be requested. There is a nominal charge; price lists will be mailed.

Tourette Syndrome Association, Inc.
Bell Plaza Building
42-20 Bell Boulevard
Bayside, NY 11361
(212) 224-2999

Handicapping Conditions Served: Gilles de la Tourette syndrome (TS).

The Organization: Established in 1972 by patients and their families, the Association offers information and moral support to others affected by this condition through its 18 chapters in the U.S., Canada, and England. Neuropsychiatric symptoms that characterize this genetic disorder appear in childhood and may be misdiagnosed for an average of 10 years, creating severe psychological damage in the patient and family. For this reason, Association activities emphasize early identification and treatment. Education of professionals as well as the general public is conducted through publications and the media to alert physicians and families to the signs and symptoms of the syndrome. Since the cause and cure are not known, the Association supports medical research by advocacy, fund raising, and solicitation of autopsy brain tissue for the Mt. Sinai Medical Center Brain Bank.

Information Services: As the only clearinghouse of information on TS, the Association maintains a current referral file of physicians throughout the country who are working with patients. Informational exhibits are held at medical conventions each year to acquaint more physicians with current research and treatment. The quarterly *TSA Newsletter* reports on medical progress throughout the world as well as on activities of local chapters. Lists of insurance companies, TS chapters, bibliographies, and article reprints for professionals and patients, membership information, and a public education film, "The Sudden Intruder," are available on request.

**United Cerebral Palsy Associations,
   Inc. (UCPA)**
66 E. 34th Street
New York, NY 10016
(212) 481-6300

Handicapping Conditions Served: Cerebral palsy and other neuromotor disabilities.

The Organization: The United Cerebral Palsy Associations' (UCPA) programs and services are directed toward a two-fold goal—the prevention of cerebral palsy, and meeting the needs of those who are affected by the conditions and others who have similar service needs. To fulfill this goal, UCPA 1) provides funds for research and the training of scientific personnel who work in the fields of prevention and treatment of cerebral palsy; 2) acts as an advocate of the civil rights of the disabled in the areas of education, employment, independent living, and access to public buildings and public transportation; 3) provides public education programs in schools, hospitals, and community facilities, which emphasize prevention of neuromotor problems; and 4) through its 256 state and local affiliates, provides direct services including: medical diagnosis, evaluation and treatment, special education, career development, social and recreational programs, parent counseling, adapted housing for the disabled, advocacy, and community education.

Information Services: Through a variety of publications as well as telephone and letter responses to inquiries, UCPA provides extensive information about the nature of cerebral palsy, the means of preventing the condition, the services available to and required by persons with cerebral palsy and their families, and the civil rights of persons with disabilities. The Association sponsors **Project Prevention**, a public education program to inform prospective mothers about how they should care for themselves in order to lessen the possibility of neuromotor problems in their babies. Vaccination of children against childhood diseases is also stressed. UCPA's **Project Prevention** Program Packet containing health education materials is available free. Additional lay publications include: *What Everyone Should Know about Cerebral Palsy*, a cartoon booklet describing the causes of the conditions, management techniques, available services, and the outlook for prevention; and a *Parent's Kit*, which emphasizes parents' roles in their child's development and the assistance they may need in coping with the problems that a disabled child presents.

In the advocacy area, UCPA publications include a bibliography on housing and the handicapped, a handbook on transportation, a report on work programs for the multihandicapped, and a report on alternative living arrangements for teenagers and adults with cerebral palsy. UCPA publishes a bimonthly general interest newsletter and issues a monthly newsletter dealing with the governmental matters of concern to the disabled. For professionals and volunteers, the Association's publications include materials on child development; testing, management, and treatment of cerebral palsy; service needs; Federal assistance programs; and fund raising. The Association holds frequent workshops for professionals which focus on upgrading the quality of patient services. Progress in the effort to prevent cerebral palsy is reported periodically in *Research Report* and *Medical Director's Report*. Most information is provided free to any inquirer.

United Ostomy Association, Inc. (UOA)
2001 W. Beverly Boulevard
Los Angeles, CA 90057
(213) 413-5510

Handicapping Conditions Served: Ileostomy, colostomy, and urinary ostomy patients.

The Organization: Formed by an alliance of 28 local chapters in 1962, the Association now has more than 550 chapters in the U.S. and Canada. Volunteers are trained to visit new patients in hospitals and offer the information and moral support that only a fellow ostomate can provide. Monthly chapter meetings as well as regional and national conferences are held at which medical professionals and patients conduct demonstrations, workshops, and equipment presentations to educate ostomates, their families, and health professionals in the management and care necessary following surgery.

Information Services: UOA publishes informational brochures explaining the surgery and postoperative care for patients. Educational materials for doctors and nurses discuss management as well as attitudes and psychological difficulties patients may develop in connection with surgery. Public information programs are conducted in an effort to eliminate job and insurance discrimination.

Publications include booklets on surgery, management and care (in English, Spanish, French, and Chinese), for patients. Fact sheets and catalogs describing insurance, equipment, and suppliers, and a quarterly magazine are available. Special problems children may have in accepting their condition, or that adults may have with personal and sexual relationships or childbearing, are dealt with in other publications—all available at nominal cost from the Association.

United Parkinson Foundation (UPF)
220 S. State Street
Chicago, IL 60604
(312) 922-9734

Handicapping Conditions Served: Parkinson's disease.

The Organization: The United Parkinson Foundation (UPF) is a membership organization for Parkinson patients and their families. UPF assembles information about the disease and disseminates it to members and nonmembers alike. UPF also gives financial assistance to researchers who are studying the disease.

Information Services: Booklets on exercise, research, and therapies are available at no cost to Parkinson patients and their families, and the information in the booklets is supplemented and updated by UPF's quarterly newsletter. The organization maintains a national list of diagnostic, treatment, and rehabilitation centers for the patient, and it can provide the names of retail outlets for obtaining prosthetic devices and special equipment. At the request of the patient, UPF will contact the patient's employer to explain Parkinson's disease and the work limitations, if any. UPF sponsors scientific symposia on Parkinson's disease for lay audiences. Professionals are permitted on-site use of UPF's collection of reprints of scientific papers. For information, contact Ms. Judy Rosner, Executive Director.

Part Two

INFORMATION/DATA BANKS

All Federal Agencies are asterisked for easy identification.

Page

Page

Accent on Information
P.O. Box 700
Bloomington, IL 61701
(309) 378-2961

Handicapping Conditions Served: All handicaps; primarily persons with physical disabilities.

The Organization: Founded in 1968, Accent on Information (AOI) is a computerized retrieval system containing information on products and devices which assist disabled persons and other how-to information in such areas as eating, bathing, grooming, clothing, furniture, home management, toilet care, sexuality, mobility, and written and oral communication. The citations in this data base, which number about 4,000, give two types of information: 1) references to publications on topics covered, including sources; and 2) brief descriptions of equipment and devices with addresses of manufacturers marketing the products.

Information Services: For a nominal charge, a search of the AOI system is made on the requestor's topic. The requestor receives up to 25 recent citations for each search.

The *Buyer's Guide*, which grew out of AOI's information retrieval system, lists equipment and devices which assist disabled persons in daily living activities. Manufacturers which market these products are also listed.

Other publications available from AOI include titles on devices and techniques for persons with the use of only one hand, accessibility in the home, home operated businesses for disabled persons, clothing, attendant care, sexuality, and bowel management for persons with spinal cord injuries. The *Accent on Living* magazine, issued quarterly, contains information on new publications, products, techniques, and civil rights for disabled persons; true life stories; and other practical and inspirational articles.

Arthritis Information Clearinghouse
P.O. Box 34427
Bethesda, MD 20034
(301) 881-9411

Handicapping Conditions Served: Arthritis, gout, SLE (systemic lupus erythematosus), bone diseases (including Paget's disease), and other musculoskeletal disorders.

The Organization: The Clearinghouse is a service of the National Institute of Arthritis, Metabolism, and Digestive Diseases, HEW, and is designed to help health professionals identify materials for professional and patient education. It was established in 1978.

Information Services: The Clearinghouse is not a distributor of materials produced elsewhere, but will refer clients to the appropriate sources. The collection focuses on 1975 and later materials, print and audiovisual. Also collected are descriptions of community demonstration projects applicable to patient education in the arthritis field; and the sources of information in that field. The data base is computerized and can produce custom bibliographies. The *Bulletin* announces availability of materials, highlights Clearinghouse resources and services, and reports on professional programs and other events. Bibliographies are available on such topics as arthritis and employment; psychological factors in arthritis; joint replacement; and juvenile rheumatoid arthritis. Brief directories on organizations and information resources and on public information materials have been prepared by the Clearinghouse. Reference sheets cover topics ranging from employment to osteoarthritis to patient education program design. Services to patients are not within the scope of the Clearinghouse.

Brain Information Service (BIS)
Center for the Health Sciences
University of California
Los Angeles, CA 90024
(213) 825-6011

Handicapping Conditions Served: Neurological disorders in general, mental/emotional disorders in general, gonadal reproductive disorders, and blindness/visual impairments.

The Organization: Established in 1964, the Brain Information Service (BIS) currently receives funding from the Office of the Director, National Institutes of Health. BIS covers the world's literature in the basic neurological sciences of neuroanatomy, neurophysiology, neurochemistry, neuroendocronology, neuropharmacology, and behavior. Information on the neurological aspects of many handicapping conditions is included.

Information Services: BIS produces serial publications geared to researchers and teachers in the neurosciences, for which there is a subscription fee. Professional inquirers may request any of the BIS publications as well as other information in their area of interest. Lay requestors receive reprints of articles on the brain.

Bureau of the Census
U.S. Department of Commerce
Washington, DC 20233
(202) 568-1200

Handicapping Conditions Served: General information on disability.

The Organization: The Bureau is a general purpose statistical agency which collects, tabulates, and publishes a wide variety of statistical data about the people and the economy of the United States. These data are utilized by Congress, by the executive branch, and by the public in the development and evaluation of economic and social programs. In addition, the Bureau conducts special censuses at the request and expense of states and local government units; publishes estimates and projections of the population; provides current data on population and housing characteristics; and issues current reports on other subjects.

Information Services: The principal products of the Bureau are its printed reports, computer tapes, and special tabulations. However, it also produces statistical compendia, catalogs, guides, and directories which are useful in locating information on specific subjects.

The following publications, which may be purchased from the Superintendent of Documents, U.S. Government Printing Office, Washington, DC 20402, are of particular interest to organizations serving disabled persons:

• *Persons with Work Disability*, which reports on 1970 Census data collected on work-related disability from a sample of five percent of the population, lists statistics on the presence and duration of work disability for the noninstitutional population 18 to 64 years old, classified by various demographic, social, and economic characteristics.

• *Demographic, Social, and Economic Profile of States: Spring 1976* gives intercensal estimates of the characteristics of the population of all states, generated from a single sample survey (the 1976 Survey of Income and Education). Among the data included in this report are statistics on the work disability status of persons 18 to 64 by state and sex.

A microdata file containing statistical information on 151,170 households, compiled from the 1976 Survey of Income and Education, allows analysis by state and larger standard metropolitan statistical areas. Questions included deal with income, public assistance, disability, and other variables. A brochure describing the content and structure of this file and how users may access it, entitled *Microdata from the Survey of Income and Education* (DAD No. 42), is available from the Subscriber Services Section, Bureau of the Census, Washington, DC 20233.

The 1980 Census will include a question on disability as related to employment and difficulty in using public transportation on a sample basis. This question will provide general data on the size and distribution of the disabled population.

Cancer Information Clearinghouse
National Cancer Institute
7910 Woodmont Avenue, Suite 1320
Bethesda, MD 20014
(301) 496-7070

Handicapping Conditions Served: Cancer.

The Organization: The Clearinghouse is a service of the National Cancer Institute's Office of Cancer Communications (see separate entry). The Clearinghouse finds, documents, stores, and abstracts health education materials for the patient, the public, and—to some extent—professionals. Also collected are references to planning, developing and managing of health education programs. Sources of material number in the thousands.

Information Services: Users of the Clearinghouse are organizations and health professionals engaged in public, patient, and professional education. Public contact is not encouraged, since the public is served through these intermediaries. Bibliographic materials cover screening and detection; cause and prevention; diagnosis and treatment; rehabilitation; and behavior (coping with cancer). The Clearinghouse does not actually disseminate materials but performs reference searches of its collection of about 6000 materials. Annotated bibliographies are available on oral cancer, skin cancer, nutrition for the cancer patient, patient education for ostomates, Spanish language materials, asbestos, smoking, breast cancer, coping with cancer, cancer information in the workplace, patient rights, and cancer treatment (patient materials). Bulletins are issued alerting users to new publications, programs, services, data bases, and audiovisual materials. Materials for professional education are collected in one area—audiovisuals—because no other information service provides this medical education service. Referrals are made for patients and the public to community services, Comprehensive Cancer Centers, and other sources. The Clearinghouse is a medium for exchange of information among the Centers, all of which provide community information. The Clearinghouse has a file of over 300 cancer education programs and can put professionals in touch with others who have started such programs. There is no charge for any Clearinghouse service.

Center for Innovation in Teaching
the Handicapped (CITH)
Dissemination and Retrieval Unit
Indiana University
2805 East 10th Street
Bloomington, IN 47401
(812) 337-5847

Handicapping Conditions Served: All handicaps.

The Organization: The Center for Innovation in Teaching the Handicapped (CITH), funded by the Bureau of Education for the Handicapped, is devoted to research, development, demonstration, and dissemination of innovative methods and materials for the training of preservice and inservice personnel who work with handicapped children in schools. The Center is currently focusing on addressing personnel training needs resulting from the Education for All Handicapped Children Act (P.L. 94-142). A number of current personnel training projects are related to mainstreaming handicapped children into regular classrooms.

Information Services: The Dissemination and Retrieval Unit of the Center is responsible for the distribution of the Center's products, which include nearly 300 CITH research reports, working documents, training packages, and printed and audiovisual training materials. Self-instructional materials for teachers of the handicapped include *Tips for Teachers Series, Instructional Development for Training Teachers of Exceptional Children, Individualized Education Programs,* and *The Hypothesis/Test Reading Program.* A directory of CITH publications and materials is available upon request.

Clearinghouse on the Handicapped
Office for Handicapped Individuals, HEW
Room 338D Hubert H. Humphrey Building
Washington, DC 20201
(202) 245-1961

This office will be transferred to the Department of Education, Office of Special Education and Rehabilitative Services within the next few months. Address changes will be announced in Programs for the Handicapped. *You may wish to request notification by sending the self-mailer card inserted in the Directory.*

Handicapping Conditions Served: All handicaps.

The Organization: The Clearinghouse on the Handicapped is part of the Office for Handicapped Individuals which has been the focus within the Office of Human Development Services and the Department for review, coordination, information and planning related to policies, programs, procedures, and activities relevant to the physically and mentally handicapped.

The Clearinghouse, besides providing direct information services, researches and monitors information operations on the national, state, and local level serving the handicapped and related personnel, and provides technical assistance to such operations on request.

Information Services: The Clearinghouse responds to inquiries on a wide range of topics concerning handicapping conditions and related services. If it cannot supply a direct answer, the inquirer is referred to relevant information sources which have been researched and with which the Clearinghouse maintains ongoing contacts. The Clearinghouse is especially knowledgeable in Federal funding for programs serving the handicapped, Federal programs and Federal legislation. Its publication program is oriented towards producing publications of use to information providers. Its publication, *Directory of National Information Sources on Handicapping Conditions and Related Services,* is an important tool in the networking of existing information operations by describing organizations with capabilities and competencies in the field.

The Clearinghouse also puts out publications on statistics, barrier-free access, recreation, and other topics. A bimonthly newsletter, *Programs for the Handicapped*, monitors activities of Federal agencies and other national organizations and announces new publications of the Clearinghouse and other sources. There is no charge for the Clearinghouse's services or publications.

Closer Look
Parents' Campaign for Handicapped
**   Children and Youth**
Box 1492
Washington, DC 20013
(202) 833-4160

Handicapping Conditions Served: All handicaps.

The Organization: Closer Look, funded under a contract with the Bureau of Education for the Handicapped, U.S. Office of Education, is a national information center for parents of handicapped children, professionals, and other persons interested in 1) the right of disabled persons to obtain educational and other services, 2) consumer advocacy and coalition building, and 3) information on national, state, and local organizations which meet the needs of handicapped persons. Established in 1970, Closer Look is operated by the Parents' Campaign for Handicapped Children and Youth, a nonprofit organization of parents who advocate for the rights of disabled children. The Campaign works closely with local parent groups throughout the country.

Closer Look has developed a large collection of written material which explain legal rights in lay language, steer parents to appropriate resources, and provide practical advice on daily living problems.

Information Services: Closer Look responds to most inquiries by sending out packets of information tailored to the requestor's information needs. Parents typically receive lists of state agencies and local parent groups, referrals to organizations serving persons with their child's disability, information on legal rights and parent advocacy, and brochures pertinent to the age group of the child. These brochures include *One Step at a Time*, a guide for parents of babies and young children whose growth is slow, unusual, or affected by a disability; *Helping the Handicapped Teenager Mature*; and fact sheets on recreation and vocational education. Booklets on testing and evaluation are also available.

Among materials sent to adult inquirers with disabilities are brochures on the rights of handicapped persons, higher education, rehabilitation, employment, housing, and recreation, and a list of voluntary organizations which disseminate information on disabilities and advocate for handicapped persons.

Information for teachers includes publications on handicapping conditions, attitudes, P.L. 94-142 and the "least restrictive environment" it mandates, and a book list for future reading.

Students interested in a teaching career may obtain information on institutions of higher education which offer training in special education.

There is no charge for Closer Look's services or publications, which include a biannual newsletter.

Requestors are asked to write rather than telephone Closer Look, since the information packets sent to inquirers contain more information than can be given over the telephone.

Conference Papers Index (CPI)
Data Courier, Inc.
620 South Fifth Street
Louisville, KY 40202
(502) 582-4111

Handicapping Conditions Served: All handicaps.

The Organization: Produced and marketed by Data Courier, Inc., Conference Papers Index (CPI) cites and indexes scientific and technical papers presented at regional, national, and international professional meetings. Some of the more than 100,000 citations added each year are not recorded elsewhere in print. Citations include titles of papers, names of authors, addresses when available, and information on how to obtain preprints, reprints, and conference publications. Main subjects covered are engineering, the physical sciences, and the life sciences (medicine, pharmacology, biochemistry, and other fields). Citations on handicapping conditions in such areas as rehabilitation medicine, facilities, and transportation are included in CPI.

Information Services: CPI is available as an online data base through Lockheed and the System Development Corporation (see Data Base Vendors, page 97), and as a monthly journal published by Data Courier. Annual indexes and back issues of the journal may also be purchased.

The Council for Exceptional Children
Information Service
1920 Association Drive
Reston, VA 22091
(800) 336-3728 (except Virginia)
(703) 620-3660 (Virginia, collect calls are accepted)

Handicapping Conditions Served: All handicaps.

The Organization: The Council for Exceptional Children (CEC), a private, nonprofit membership organization, was established in 1922 to advance the education of exceptional children and youth, both handicapped and gifted. CEC Information Services acts as an information broker for teachers, administrators, students, parents, and others, serving as a comprehensive literature depository for English language materials. The ERIC Clearinghouse on Handicapped and Gifted Children, housed at CEC, catalogs, indexes, and abstracts journal articles and research reports for inclusion in the ERIC data base (see separate entry).

CEC has developed an in-house data base, Exceptional Child Education Resources (ECER), which began in 1969 as an abstract journal. This file contains documents entered into ERIC by the Clearinghouse on Handicapped and Gifted Children (approximately 50% of ECER records) and special education materials not appropriate to the ERIC system, such as textbooks, doctoral dissertations in special education, journals not scanned for ERIC, and nonprint media for use in professional training programs. ECER, which contains bibliographic data and abstracts on approximately 40,000 documents, has been searchable on-line since 1971.

The Policy Research Center of the CEC Governmental Relations Unit monitors and analyzes policies concerning exceptional children, conducts policy research in this area, and works to encourage policies favorable to the development of exceptional persons. This Center maintains a reference library of policy information on handicapped and gifted persons, included Federal, state, and local laws, regulations, guidelines, litigation, and policy reports.

In addition, CEC's twelve divisions, which focus on particular aspects of special education, are autonomous in developing professional programs and publications geared to meet the needs of division members. These divisions are (periodicals available to non-members by subscription are listed in parenthesis): Council of Administrators of Special Education Incorporated, Council for Children with Behavioral Disorders (*Behavioral Disorders*); Division on Mental Retardation (*Education and Training of the Mentally Retarded*); Council for Educational Diagnostic Services (*Diagnostique**); Division on Career Development (*Career Development for Exceptional Individuals**), Division for Children with Communication Disorders, Division for Children with Learning Disabilities (*Learning Disability Quarterly*); Division on Early Childhood, Division on Physically Handicapped, Division for the Visually Handicapped, Association for the Gifted (*Journal for the Education of the Gifted*); and Teacher Education Division (*Teacher Education and Special Education*). An asterisk (*) indicates that subscriptions are available to libraries only.

Information Services: Custom computer searches of the ECER, ERIC and other education oriented data bases are available from CEC for a charge. Reprints of previous searches or selected popular topics may also be ordered. In Addition, current awareness service offers subscribers printouts containing the newest ECER citations and abstracts in custom-designed subject areas eight times per year.

CEC produces numerous publications on special education, awareness of handicapped people, child abuse, recreation, parent-professional cooperation, career and vocational education, severely handicapped children, and public policy. Bibliographies on topics of current interest and nonprint media are also available. In addition, subscriptions to the ECER journal, which appears quarterly, may be ordered.

Original documents or microfiche copies of most ECER documents are retained in CEC's library, which also houses over 250 periodicals, the complete ERIC microfiche collection, and many reference materials. The library is open to the public Monday through Friday.

The Policy Research Center (PRC), described above, provides information, consultation, and technical assistance on special education policy to persons, groups, and agencies. Inquiries requiring PRC research are accommodated on a contract basis; PRC acceptance of contract work depends on the availability of staff time and CEC policy and priorities.

CEC Information Services responds to thousands of requests each year from professionals, students, parents, and others. When appropriate, inquirers are referred to other organizations. Users are asked not to direct inquiries to both CEC and the ERIC Clearinghouse on Handicapped and Gifted Children, since the two organizations share staff and resources in responding to requests.

The ECER data base may be accessed directly through Bibliographic Retrieval Service and Lockheed (See Data Base Vendors, page 97).

CRISP
Statistics and Analysis Branch
Division of Research Grants
National Institute of Health, NIH
Bethesda, MD 20205
(301) 496-7543

Handicapping Conditions Served: All handicaps.

The Organization: The mission of the Statistics and Analysis Branch in the Division of Research Grants at the National Institutes of Health (NIH) includes the operation of a large computer-based information system, Computer Retrieval of Information on Scientific Projects (CRISP), developed to facilitate the rapid dissemination of current scientific information on research projects supported through the various research grants and contracts programs of the Public Health Service or conducted intramurally by NIH and the National Institute of Mental Health. On the basis of applications or progress reports for extramural research, and annual reports or project narratives for intramural research, awarded projects are indexed by NIH staff scientists. The file contains approximately 500,000 items, many of which report on research on disabling diseases and conditions, including the following: cerebral palsy, mental retardation, spina bifida and other congenital abnormalities, blindness, deafness, metabolic disorders, multiple sclerosis and other diseases of the nervous system, spinal cord injuries, amputation, mental illness, and all other major handicapping conditions.

Information Services: CRISP will perform searches of the data base on single specific topics (e.g., sickle cell disease) or generic data (e.g., all research support on cancer). The computer printout includes information on the research area, disease, materials, and methods. For routine searches, there is no charge to government agencies, public interest groups, other nonprofit organizations, and individuals; profit-making organizations must pay for searches.

Dissertation Information Services
University Microfilms International
300 N. Zeeb Road
Ann Arbor, MI 48106
(313) 761-4700
(800) 521-3042 (for ordering and information)

Handicapping Conditions Served: All handicaps.

The Organization: University Microfilms International (UMI) was founded in 1938 to provide researchers with difficult-to-obtain books and articles. Its publications include books, periodicals, and monographs, which are printed, photocopied, or microfilmed. UMI also operates information retrieval systems for its publication programs. The company's Dissertation Information Services allow access to the more than 600,000 published dissertations accepted at North American colleges and universities. Recently this program has been broadened to include some foreign universities.

Information Services: Customers may order searches of the Comprehensive Dissertation Index (CDI), UMI's data base of references to published dissertations in 77 major subject and 119 minor subject areas. Computer printouts delivered to the user include the dissertation title, author, publication date, degree, subject field, school, and for dissertations published by UMI, the page and volume reference to *Dissertation Abstracts International* (DAI), a UMI monthly publication giving concise author-prepared summaries of dissertations. CDI contains more than 4,000 records of deafness, blindness, mental retardation, birth defects, special education, rehabilitation, and other disabling conditions and related services.

Users may also consult a publication issued periodically, the *Comprehensive Dissertation Index*, which gives bibliographic information on almost every doctoral dissertation accepted in North America since 1861. For those titles published by UMI, a reference to the DAI location is included. Subject bibliographies and catalogs of dissertations and theses on topics of widespread interest are available to librarians and researchers at no charge.

Free copies of *The Researchers Guide to Dissertation Information Services*, which describes the full line of the company's dissertation-related services and products, are available.

Users with computer terminals may access CDI directly through arrangements with Bibliographic Retrieval Services, Lockheed, or the System Development Corporation (See Data Base Vendors, page 97).

Educational Resources Information Center
Central ERIC
National Institute of Education, HEW
Washington, DC 20208
(202) 254-5500

Handicapping Conditions Served: All handicaps.

The Organization: ERIC is a decentralized nationwide network, sponsored by the National Institute of Education and designed to collect educational documents and to make them available to teachers, administrators, researchers, students, and other interested persons. ERIC is made up of 16 clearinghouses located across the country, each specializing in a particular subject area of education. The exact number of clearinghouses has fluctuated over time in response to the shifting needs of the educational community. Central ERIC provides the funding for the clearinghouses and document processing operations, sets policies, and monitors the overall functioning of the information system.

The clearinghouses are responsible for collecting all relevant unpublished, noncopyrighted or copyright released materials of value in their subject areas. These include current research findings, project and technical reports, speeches and unpublished manuscripts, conference proceedings, books, and professional journal articles. At the clearinghouses these items are screened according to ERIC selection criteria, abstracted, and indexed. All of this information is entered in a central ERIC computer data base and announced in the ERIC reference publications.

Information Services: All documents entered into the ERIC system are listed in the following periodicals:

• *Resources in Education* (RIE), a monthly abstract journal announcing recently completed research reports, descriptions of outstanding programs, other documents of educational significance, indexed by subject, author, and institutional source. Cumulative semiannual indexes are available. RIE may be ordered from the Superintendent of Documents, U.S. Government Printing Office, Washington, DC 20402.

• *Current Index to Journals in Education* (CIJE), a monthly guide to the periodical literature, with

58

coverage of more than 700 major educational and education-related publications. It includes a main entry section with annotations, and is indexed by subject, author, and journal title. Annual cumulative indexes are available. Subscriptions to CIJE are available from Oryx Press, 2214 N. Central Avenue, Phoenix, AZ 85004.

The ERIC Document Reproduction Service (EDRS), operated by Computer Microfilm International Corporation, 3030 N. Fairfax Drive, Suite 200, Arlington, VA 22201, (703) 841-1212, produces microfiche and paper copies of most documents announced in RIE. Over 650 institutions and organizations, including many libraries, receive complete sets of ERIC documents on microfiche. Sources for items included in RIE and not available from EDRS are given in the RIE listing.

Copies of articles from a majority of journals regularly covered in CIJE are available through a reprint service from University Microfilms International, 300 N. Zeeb Road, Ann Arbor, MI 48106.

In addition to searching the ERIC reference publications, which are available in many libraries, researchers may obtain custom searches of the ERIC data base. These are available from each clearinghouse (see entries for the following ERIC Clearinghouses: Adult, Career and Vocational Education; Handicapped and Gifted Children; Reading and Communication Skills; Teacher Education; and Tests, Measurement, and Evaluation.) (ERIC Clearinghouses with less relevance to special education and therefore not covered in this Directory are listed below.) Searches may also be obtained from one of the libraries, agencies, and other organizations which have access to this file. There are advantages in contacting the ERIC clearinghouse that has responsibility for processing documents in the inquirier's specific area of interest: 1) the information specialists at each clearinghouse are knowledgeable about the contents of the data base in the clearinghouse's subject area, and are therefore able to formulate effective search strategies; and 2) each clearinghouse has a number of products in its subject area which it disseminates to its users, i.e., short bibliographies, resource lists and newsletters.

Access points for computerized ERIC searches are listed in the *Directory of ERIC Search Services*, available at no charge from the ERIC Processing and Reference Facility, 4833 Rugby Avenue, Suite 303, Bethesda, MD 20014. Some of these centers serve only specific user groups; others have no restrictions on clientele. Cost per search and turn-around time vary with each center.

Authors of reports, speeches, papers, etc., who would like to have their materials considered for national dissemination through ERIC may forward their contributions to the ERIC Processing and Reference Facility, Information Systems Division, 4833 Rugby Avenue, Suite 303, Bethesda, MD 20014. Documents are forwarded to the proper clearinghouse, screened, and if found appropriate, entered into the ERIC system.

The ERIC data base is available commercially through Bibliographic Retrieval Services, Lockheed, and the System Development Corporation (see Data Base Vendors, page 97).

Other ERIC Clearinghouses:

ERIC Clearinghouse on Educational Management
University of Oregon
Eugene, OR 97403
(503) 686-5043

ERIC Clearinghouse on Higher Education
George Washington University
One Dupont Circle, Suite 630
Washington, DC 20036
(202) 296-2597

ERIC Clearinghouse on Information Resources
Syracuse University
School of Education
Syracuse, NY 13210
(315) 423-3640

ERIC Clearinghouse for Junior Colleges
University of California
Powell Library, Room 96
Los Angeles, CA 90024
(213) 825-3931

ERIC Clearinghouse on Languages
    and Linguistics
Center for Applied Linguistics
1611 North Kent Street
Arlington, VA 22209
(703) 528-4312

ERIC Clearinghouse on Rural Education and
   Small Schools
New Mexico State University
Box 3AP
Las Cruces, NM 88003
(505) 646-2623

ERIC Clearinghouse for Science, Mathematics,
   and Environmental Education
Ohio State University
1200 Chambers Road, Third Floor
Columbus, OH 43212
(614) 422-6717

ERIC Clearinghouse for Social Studies/Social
   Science Education
855 Broadway
Boulder, CO 80302
(303) 492-8434

ERIC Clearinghouse on Urban Education
Box 40
Teachers College
Columbia University
525 W. 120th Street
New York, NY 10027
(212) 678-3437

**ERIC Clearinghouse on Adult, Career
   and Vocational Education
The National Center for Research
   in Vocational Education
The Ohio State University
1960 Kenny Road
Columbus, OH 43210
(614) 486-3655**

Handicapping Conditions Served: All handicaps.

The Organization: The scope of the ERIC Clearinghouse on Adult, Career, and Vocational Education encompasses the following areas: 1) adult and continuing education—including adult basic education, educational gerontology, community education and development, and professional skill upgrading; 2) career education—including career awareness, exploration and development, prevocational education, career centers, and experience-based career education; 3) vocational and technical education—including agricultural education, business and office education, health education, home economics, trade and industrial education, and new vocational and technical fields; and 4) education and work—including comprehensive employment and training, youth employment, school-to-work transition, job training and placement, and apprenticeships. Information on disabled persons is available in many of these subject areas.

Information Services: The Clearinghouse provides publications and user services, including custom searches of the ERIC data base described above. Bibliographies and resource lists on topics of current interest, including career education and individualized education programs for handicapped students, are additional Clearinghouse services. The Clearinghouse's information analysis series is designed to assist teachers, administrators, researchers, and other educational practitioners by providing reviews, analyses, syntheses, and interpretations of current literature in selected subject areas. A few of the titles in this publication series are of interest to professionals working with disabled persons. The Clearinghouse also publishes information bulletins on a periodic basis to highlight ERIC materials, products, and activities.

The Clearinghouse staff provides consultation on information search problems and, when appropriate, refers clients to additional educational resources. There is a charge for some services and publications, including computer searches of the ERIC data base.

The ERIC data base is available commercially through Bibliographic Retrieval Services, Lockheed, and the System Development Corporation (see Data Base Vendors, page 97).

**ERIC Clearinghouse for Counseling
and Personnel Services**
2108 School of Education
University of Michigan
Ann Arbor, MI 48109
(313) 764-9492

Handicapping Conditions Served: All handicaps.

The Organization: The ERIC Clearinghouse for Counseling and Personnel Services (CAPS) focuses on resources for the professional. Information relating to the continuing education of helping services personnel include the following subject areas: counselor training, development, and evaluation; student characteristics and environments; family relationships; career planning; drug education and abuse; and special populations such as women, youth, dropouts, aged, incarcerated, widowed and divorced, and handicapped. (Information on career education for disabled persons is available from the ERIC Clearinghouse on Adult, Career, and Vocational Education; see separate entry.)

Information Services: CAPS offers computer searches of ERIC and other data bases relevant to the counseling and prescribed fields. The cost varies according to the data base selected.

CAPS puts out a variety of publications, including the *Cumulative Index of ERIC Resources in Counseling and Personnel Services*, monographs on specific issues in the helping services, and *Searchlights*, which are computer produced bibliographies on topics of current interest. *Counseling the Exceptional: Handicapped and Gifted*, Searchlight 32+, contains an article on the state-of-the-art in counseling services for handicapped and gifted persons and an annotated listing of over 150 references on the subject. A new publication, *Counseling Exceptional People*, describes practical counseling techniques to use with specific disabilities and giftedness. There is a nominal charge for CAPS publications.

CAPS conducts national, state, and local workshops on topics of current educational interest, also designed to familiarize participants with ERIC tools and materials. The CAPS Learning Resources Center, open to the public, houses the complete ERIC collection, and professional books, journals, newsletters, and magazines on helping services.

The ERIC data base is available commercially through Bibliographic Retrieval Services, Lockheed, and the System Development Corporation (see Data Base Vendors, page 97).

**ERIC Clearinghouse on Elementary
and Early Childhood Education**
College of Education
University of Illinois
Urbana, IL 61801
(217) 333-1386

Handicapping Conditions Served: All handicaps.

The Organization: The ERIC Clearinghouse on Elementary and Early Childhood Education collects documents about child development and behavior from the prenatal period through age 12, day care, early childhood education, and general aspects of elementary education. Material on mainstreaming falls within the scope of the Clearinghouse. Specific curriculum areas and related fields (such as testing, counseling, and administration) are handled by other ERIC clearinghouses (see separate entries).

Information Services: Searches of the ERIC data base, resource lists, bibliographies, papers on topics of current interest, and a newsletter are available from the Clearinghouse. Publications of interest to special educators include *Teaching the Special Child in Regular Classrooms* and lists of recent resources on handicapped children and children's health. Referrals are made to other organizations when appropriate. There is a charge for ERIC searches and some publications.

The ERIC data base is available commercially through Bibliographic Retrieval Services, Lockheed, and the System Development Corporation (see Data Base Vendors, page 97).

**ERIC Clearinghouse on Handicapped
    and Gifted Children
Council for Exceptional Children
1920 Association Drive
Reston, VA 22091
(800) 336-3738 (Except Virginia)
(703) 620-3660 (Virginia, collect calls are accepted)**

Handicapping Conditions Served: All handicaps.

The Organization: Housed at the Council for Exceptional Children (CEC), (see separate entry), the ERIC Clearinghouse on Handicapped and Gifted Children processes documents on research, programs, evaluation methods, administration, services, teacher education, and curricula related to handicapped and gifted children and youth.

Information Services: Searches of the ERIC data base, Exceptional Child Education Resources (an in-house data base developed at CEC and described under the entry for CEC), and other files relevant to education may be ordered from the Clearinghouse. In addition, the Clearinghouse publishes: 1) fact sheets and brief bibliographies on topics of current interest; 2) a newsletter; and 3) information analysis products, which are books and monographs focusing on emerging trends or research analysis, produced jointly with CEC. There is a charge for computer searches and for most publications.

Users are asked not to direct inquiries to both CEC and the Clearinghouse, since there is considerable overlap between CEC Information Services, which handles information requests, and the Clearinghouse.

The ERIC data base is available commercially through Bibliographic Retrieval Services, Lockheed, and the System Development Corporation (see Data Base Vendors, page 97).

**ERIC Clearinghouse on Reading
    and Communication Skills
National Council of Teachers of English
1111 Kenyon Road
Urbana, IL 61801
(217) 328-3870**

Handicapping Conditions Served: Communication and language disorders.

The Organization: The ERIC Clearinghouse on Reading and Communication Skills collects, analyzes, and disseminates educational information on the language arts and related disciplines. The Clearinghouse is concerned with all dimensions on human communication, especially with the acquisition of functional competence in reading, writing, speaking, and listening at all educational levels and in all social contexts. The placement of handicapped students in regular arts programs and the development of communications skills in the learning disabled are areas covered by the Clearinghouse.

Information Services: The Clearinghouse provides searches of the ERIC data base and copies of journal articles, books, reports, booklets, extensive bibliographies, and mini-bibliographies on subjects within the scope of the Clearinghouse. Copies of an article entitled "Mainstreaming and Reading Instruction," and mini-bibliographies on mainstreaming and reading and on learning disabilities are available from the Clearinghouse. There is a charge for searches and for most publications.

The ERIC data base is available commercially through Bibliographic Retrieval Services, Lockheed, and the System Development Corporation (see Data Base Vendors, page 97).

ERIC Clearinghouse on Teacher Education
One Dupont Circle, Suite 616
Washington, DC 20036
(202) 293-7280

Handicapping Conditions Served: All handicaps.

The Organization: The ERIC Clearinghouse on Teacher Education specializes in education personnel preparation, health education, physical education, recreation education, and teacher preparation for mainstreaming.

Information Services: The Clearinghouse provides searches of the ERIC data base; information analysis products, which synthesize ERIC literature on selected topics within the scope of the Clearinghouse; current issues publications on emerging trends; and annotated bibliographies of materials in the ERIC file. Among the information analysis products of interest to special educators are: *Teacher Centers as an Approach to Staff Development in Special Education, Humanizing Preservice Teacher Education: Strategies for Alcohol and Drug Abuse Prevention,* and *P.L. 94-142 Reaches the Classroom.* There is a charge for searches and for most publications.

The ERIC data base is available commercially through Bibliographic Retrieval Services, Lockheed, and the System Development Corporation (see Data Base Vendors, page 97).

ERIC Clearinghouse on Tests,
    Measurements, and Evaluation
Education Testing Service
Princeton, NJ 08541
(609) 921-9000

Handicapping Conditions Served: All handicaps.

The Organization: The ERIC Clearinghouse on Tests, Measurement, and Evaluation processes documents in the following areas of interest: 1) tests or other measurement devices; 2) measurement or evaluation procedures and techniques; 3) human development (documents concerned only with infancy and early childhood are not within the scope of the Clearinghouse); and 4) learning theory in general. Documents on subject-referenced learning (i.e., mathematics or language), or learning patterns in specific populations (i.e., handicapped or disadvantaged) are handled by other ERIC clearinghouses (see separate listings).

Information Services: The Clearinghouse staff assists inquirers by providing information on the ERIC system, by assisting in the preparation of search strategies, and by searching the ERIC data base to prepare customized bibliographies. There is a charge for ERIC searches.

The Clearinghouse has produced a number of publications on testing and evaluation, including annotated bibliographies on measures of drug knowledge, use and abuse; developmental scales for use with normal and handicapped preschool children; tests for the deaf and hearing impaired; tests of the brain damaged; tests for the mentally retarded; identification of learning disabilities; tests for the physically handicapped; nonverbal aptitude tests; vocational measures appropriate for the handicapped; and attitudes toward the handicapped. There is a charge for bibliographies and for most other Clearinghouse publications.

The ERIC data base is available commercially through Bibliographic Retrieval Services, Lockheed, and the System Development Corporation (see Data Base Vendors, page 97).

Excerpta Medica, Inc.
P.O. Box 3085
Princeton, NJ 08540
(609) 896-9450

Handicapping Conditions Served: All handicaps.

The Organization: Excerpta Medica, a comprehensive index of medical literature, was founded in 1946 with the aim of making available to medical and related professions information on all significant basic research and clinical findings reported in any language throughout the world. Since 1972, Excerpta Medica has been part of Elsevier, a major scientific publishing group with headquarters in Amsterdam, The Netherlands.

Information Services: The main product of Excerpta Medica is a series of more than 40 abstract journals covering specialized subjects in biomedical and related fields. Rehabilitation medicine, epilepsy, and drug dependence are areas of particular strength. Articles from more than 3,500 journals from 110 countries are indexed. Since 1968, these abstract journals have been produced by a computer system which has made possible automated retrieval and dissemination of information.

On-line access to the Excerpta Medica base from June 1974 to present (over a million records) is available through Lockheed Information Systems. Off-line searches of earlier records (from 1973) may be ordered from Excerpta Medica, P.O. Box 1126, 1000 BC Amsterdam, The Netherlands.

Handicapped Learner Materials
    Distribution Center (HLMDC)
Audio-Visual Center
Indiana University
Bloomington, IN 47405
(812) 337-0531

Handicapping Conditions Served: All handicaps.

The Organization: The Center is a project of the Bureau of Education for the Handicapped, Division of Media Services. The Center supplements audiovisual materials available for the handicapped student by loaning materials for direct classroom use, when these materials are not available through local, regional or state sources.

Information Services: An extensive list of audiovisual products is available, including films, videotapes, games, and adaptive devices. The Center's collection is comprised of teacher training materials (largely 16 mm films) and classroom curriculum materials for group use and individualized instruction. Video duplication services are also available. Any educator of handicapped children may request the catalogs and materials; materials are available for evaluation and/or examination. A monthly newsletter containing information about instructional materials for the handicapped is available to all clients. Other than expenses incurred by videotape duplication, HLMDC does not charge for its services.

High Blood Pressure Information
    Center
National High Blood Pressure
    Education Program
120/80 National Institutes of Health
Bethesda, MD 20205
(301) 652-7700

Handicapping Conditions Served: High blood pressure (hypertension).

The Organization: Coordinated by the National Heart, Lung and Blood Institute, National Institutes of Health, the National High Blood Pressure Education Program (NHBPEP) was begun in 1972 to reduce illness and death from hypertension by educating professionals and the public. The High Blood Pressure Information Center, operated for the Institute by Kappa Systems, is a major component of NHBPEP's professional and public education effort. The Center serves as a national clearinghouse for the collection, evaluation, and dissemination of information on hypertension.

Information Services: NHBPEP provides technical assistance to national and local agencies and organizations in a variety of ways. The Program works with health care providers to improve professional standards and guidelines for patient care and the education of practitioners. NHBPEP also reviews current patient care practices and hypertension education programs.

Services of the High Blood Pressure Information Center include reference and research assistance to health professionals and the public and the dissemination of fact sheets, reports, bibliographies, catalogs, and educational materials produced by NHBPEP and other federal and private groups. The Center maintains a roster of speakers available to address professional groups on a variety of topics related to hypertension. There is no charge for the Center's services or publications.

Highway Research Information Services (HRIS)
Transportation Research Board
2101 Constitution Avenue, N.W.
Washington, DC 20418
(202) 389-6358

Handicapping Conditions Served: Primarily physical handicaps.

The Organization: Developed by the Transportation Research Board (TRB), National Academy of Sciences, with financial support from the state highway and transportation departments and the Federal Highway Administration, the Highway Research Information Service (HRIS) is a computer based information storage and retrieval system. This file contains bibliographic information, including abstracts on articles, books, reports, and summaries of ongoing research projects from more than 1000 U.S. and foreign sources, among which are Engineering Index, the National Technical Information Service, the Smithsonian Science Information Exchange, and the U.S. Department of Transportation. There are more than 82,000 records in the file on administration, planning, design, forecasting, finance, user needs, law, safety, vehicles, and other topics. Material on the transportation of disabled persons includes the design of buses and other vehicles which accommodate handicapped persons, transportation programs for special populations, and street crossing and signal systems.

Information Services: Inquiries may obtain custom searches of the HRIS data base. Only material entered in the file since January 1970 is searched, unless the requestor asks that older material be included. The TRB staff also supplies referrals and supplemental material, including TRB publications. HRIS current awareness service provides monthly printouts of recent additions to the data base in standard subject areas and on custom-designed topics.

In addition, HRIS publishes *HRIS Abstracts*, a quarterly publication containing informative abstracts of journal articles, research reports, and technical papers and announcements of bibliographies on U.S. and foreign research.

There is a charge for HRIS searches and publications.

The HRIS data base and other transportation-related material may be accessed through TRIS-ON-LINE, a data base available from Lockheed (see Data Base Vendors, page 97).

HUD User
P.O. Box 280
Germantown, MD 20767
(301) 428-3105

Handicapping Conditions Served: All handicaps.

The Organization: Established in 1978, HUD User is an information service operated for the Office of the Assistant Secretary for Policy Development and Research (PD&R), Department of Housing and Urban Development, by Aspen Systems. PD&R is responsible for undertaking programs of research, testing, and demonstrating related to housing and community development.

The HUD User data base contains bibliographic information, including abstracts, on PD&R reports and on studies conducted by PD&R contractors. Among the subject areas covered by the file are building technology; community development; economic development and public finance; and energy and utilities. Some of the material is on barrier-free access and the housing needs of elderly and handicapped persons.

Information Services: Personalized searches of the HUD User data base are available, and printouts contain information on how to obtain copies of documents.

The *Compendium*, a semiannual annotated catalog of PD&R sponsored research results, includes descriptions of publications on handicapped-related programs and research. *Recent Research Results*, a bimonthly bulletin announcing PD&R research reports, at times includes information on studies related to disabled persons.

While most of the publications announced in the above periodicals and contained in the HUD User data base are geared to professionals, titles on energy conservation, housing needs, and other high interest areas are designed for lay persons. Copies of many documents may be obtained at no cost from HUD User. Others must be purchased from the Government Printing Office or the National Technical Information Service (separate entry). There is no charge for HUD User services or publications.

Information and Research Utilization
    Center (IRUC)
American Alliance for Health, Physical
    Education, Recreation, and Dance
    (AAHPERD)
1201 16th Street, N.W.
Washington, DC 20036
(202) 833-5547

Handicapping Conditions Served: All handicaps.

The Organization: The Information and Research Utilization Center (IRUC) was funded by the Bureau of Education for the Handicapped in 1972 as a demonstration project to collect, review, interpret, evaluate, catalog, package, and disseminate information about physical education, recreation, and related activity areas involving disabled persons. Since July 1976, IRUC has functioned as a self-supporting information center within AAHPERD's Unit on Programs for the Handicapped.

Information Services: The Center collects information and materials from programs and activities conducted in various settings, such as public and private schools, residential facilities, parks and recreation departments, and university training programs. IRUC's resource files include books, periodicals, program descriptions, audiovisual materials, curriculum guides, and listings of individuals working in areas related to physical education and recreation for the disabled. There is a charge for most services; customers include physical education and adapted physical education teachers, recreation and therapeutic recreation specialists, regular and special education classroom teachers, administrators, paraprofessionals, parents, and students. Services include:

- Publications—dealing with planning, organizing, conducting, and evaluating general and specific physical education, recreation, sports, and related activities involving handicapped persons.

- Reprint Services—of unpublished and previously published, but hard to find materials, such as curriculum guides, bibliographies, program descriptions, research reports, and demonstration projects.

- Consultation and Customized Searches—available to agencies to assist them in obtaining information for specific problems and projects.

- Referrals—to programs, program personnel, and state contacts from IRUC's computerized listings.

- *Practical Pointers*—focus on a variety of special classroom activities geared for the handicapped student.

- *Topical Updates* and *Topical Information Sheets*—information and summaries about materials dealing with topics of high interest to personnel. Examples of topics are competitive athletic programs, sex education, and liability insurance.

- *IRUC Briefings*—a newsletter including information about programs, activities, methods, research, legislation, and other areas of interest to personnel.

Information Exchange Program
Arkansas Rehabilitation Research
    and Training Center
(ARR&TC) RT-13
Hot Springs Rehabilitation Center
P.O. Box 1358
Hot Springs, AR 71901

Handicapping Conditions Served: All handicaps.

The Organization: Established in 1976 and funded by the Department of Health, Education, and Welfare, the Information Exchange Program collects materials concerning the activities of Rehabilitation Service Administration sponsored research and training centers, model spinal cord injury systems, regional rehabilitation research institutes, rehabilitation engineering centers, and the Helen Keller National Center for Deaf-Blind Youths and Adults. Information is disseminated to rehabilitation research organizations to keep the rehabilitation community aware of the latest developments and to prevent duplication of effort.

Information Services: The Program publishes the *Informer*, a quarterly journal which includes an RTC Training Calendar; the annual *Research Directory of the Rehabilitation Research and Training Center*; and a tri-annual *Publications and Audiovisual Aids Directory of the Rehabilitation Research and Training Centers*, with supplements annually.

All Program publications are free to rehabilitation professionals; as copies are available, they may be requested by other professional groups or consumers who are interested in the rehabilitation field.

Institute for Child Behavior Research
4157 Adams Avenue
San Diego, CA 92116
(714) 281-7165

Handicapping Conditions Served: Childhood psychoses, particularly childhood schizophrenia and autism.

The Organization: Founded in 1967, the Institute for Child Behavior Research conducts research on childhood schizophrenia and autism. Ongoing projects include: investigation of adequate diagnostic methods; the study of biochemical defects in autistic children; vitamin B-6 as a treatment for autism; and operant conditioning as a method of teaching autistic and schizophrenic children.

Information Services: The Institute maintains a library of detailed case studies of about 7000 children from 37 countries. Information from these computerized files is available to researchers; a fee is charged for extensive searches. The Institute has compiled a comprehensive "Diagnostic Check List for Behavior-Disturbed Children." Copies of these forms are disseminated free to institutions and private practitioners, upon request.

A summary of the reports of 3000 parents regarding the comparative effectiveness of drugs, psychotherapy, megavitamins, operant conditioning, and other forms of treatment has been published by the Institute. A periodic newsletter informs researchers, physicians, educators and parents of the latest research findings. The Institute is preparing to publish an international newsletter for information exchange among researchers throughout the world. Reprints of professional articles on childhood schizophrenia and autism may be ordered from the Institute's publications list.

Institute for Scientific Information (ISI)
325 Chestnut Street
Philadelphia, PA 19106
(215) 923-3300

Handicapping Conditions Served: All handicaps.

The Organization: ISI produces a full line of information services in the sciences, social sciences, and arts and humanities. A major portion of the world's journal literature in the physical and social sciences is indexed according to: 1) citations, based on the concept that an author's references to previously published materials indicate a subject relationship between the author's paper and earlier citations in the bibliography; 2) subject, by means of permuted title words (with each significant word in the title serving as an index term); 3) source, allowing access to records according to author; and 4) the organizational affiliation of the author.

Information Services: The *Social Science Citation Index (SSCI)*, a search tool for social sciences literature employs the indexing techniques described above. *SSCI* indexes over 130,000 items from more than 1500 journals and chapters from over 200 multi-authored books. In addition, more than 2,900 science journals are scanned for articles relevant to the social sciences. *SSCI* is issued twice a year and cumulated annually. Custom searches of the Social Scisearch data base, which allows computer retrieval of *SSCI* records, may be ordered through ISI. Most of the articles referenced, including those on handicapping conditions, are on very specific topics connected with the research of the author(s). Major disabilities, rehabilitation, and special education are represented in this file.

The *Index to Social Sciences and Humanities Proceedings*, published quarterly and cumulated annually, is a reference tool giving bibliographic information on approximately 20,000 papers each year on sociology, psychology, education, and other disciplines.

The Social Scisearch data base may be accessed through Bibliographic Retrieval Services, Lockheed, and the System Development Corporation (see Data Base Vendors, page 97).

Materials Development Center (MDC)
Stout Vocational Rehabilitation Institute
School of Education and Human Services
University of Wisconsin-Stout
Menomonie, WI 54751
(715) 232-1342

Handicapping Conditions Served: All handicaps.

The Organization: Funded in part by the Rehabilitation Services Administration, Department of Health, Education, and Welfare, the Materials Development Center (MDC) is a national central source for the collection, development, and dissemination of information and materials in the areas of vocational (work) evaluation, work adjustment, and facility management. MDC houses a comprehensive collection of publications and audiovisuals on such topics as work adjustment training, behavior modification, comparison of existing vocational evaluation systems, and rehabilitation workshop management. The Center monitors needs of professionals in these areas and conducts searches for materials which meet those needs. When suitable materials cannot be found, MDC develops, field tests, and disseminates products in the form of publications, slide/tape series, videotapes, and motion pictures.

Information Services: MDC publications and documents from other sources are listed in *Suggested Publications for Developing an Agency Library on Work Evaluation, Adjustment, and Facility Management*, available at no charge from the Center. Free brochures describe slide/tape presentations, filmstrips, cassettes, 16 mm films, and videotape and cassette recordings of national and state rehabilitation conferences. These audiovisuals may be rented or purchased from the Center. With the exception of the 16 mm films, which must be rented or purchased, personnel from state vocational rehabilitation agencies and facilities which deliver evaluation and/or adjustment services to state clients may borrow materials free of charge. Persons who meet these eligibility criteria may request searches of the MDC collection of publications and audiovisuals for information on a particular topic.

Work Sample Manual Clearinghouse Catalog, available upon request, describes MDC's work sample manuals, designed to assess the ability to perform various types of mechanical and clerical tasks. The approximate cost of assessment tools is given. State vocational rehabilitation personnel involved in vocational adjustment and work evaluation services, and rehabilitation facilities providing these services, may obtain the manuals on a free loan basis for review and possible duplication. Other facilities may rent the manuals for a nominal charge.

A free bimonthly newsletter describes MDC materials and services, as well as publications and products on evaluation, adjustment, and facility management available from other sources. There are no eligibility requirements for those who subscribe to the newsletter.

Mental Health Materials Center (MHMC)
30 East 29th Street
New York, NY 10016
(212) 889-5670

Handicapping Conditions Served: Mental and emotional disorders.

The Organization: The Mental Health Materials Center's primary objective is to facilitate the effective dissemination and utilization of publications, audiovisuals and other program aids in mental health and family life education. MHMC staff members review approximately 1,000 new pamphlets, books, films, videotapes and other audiovisuals each year for inclusion in its publications. MHMC provides consultation to agencies conducting studies relating to program materials, evaluation studies and preparation of publications.

Information Services: Professionals and para-professionals in mental health are the primary target group of MHMC. It will answer some questions for the general public; however, handicapped individuals are not directly served. Fees are charged for publications and for most research and consultative services. Organizational brochures are provided free to professionals.

MHMC's publications include a biannually updated two volume reference work: *The Selective Guide to Audiovisuals and Publications for Mental Health and Family Life Education.* To augment and update the information provided in the Guide, three quarterly newsletters are available on a subscription basis under the umbrella title *Current Information Service.*

The newsletters are: *In-Depth Reports*, covering innovative projects and programs in mental health education; *Sneak Previews*, brief evaluative reviews of all audiovisuals seen by MHMC staff and advisors; and *News, Notes and Ideas*, containing reviews of new publications and news items of interest to mental health educators.

National Arts and the Handicapped
    Information Service
Arts and Special Constituencies Project
National Endowment for the Arts
2401 E Street, N.W.
Washington, DC 20506
(202) 634-4284 (voice)
(202) 634-4138 (TTY)

Handicapping Conditions Served: All handicaps.

The Organization: The National Endowment for the Arts is a component of the National Foundation on the Arts and the Humanities, an independent agency of the Federal Government, which was created in 1965 to encourage the advancement of the nation's cultural resources. The Endowment receives an annual appropriation from Congress and is also authorized to solicit and accept private donations.

The National Arts and the Handicapped Information Service, an information and referral center, is concerned with the implementation of Section 504 of the Rehabilitation Act of 1973 in arts programs. It disseminates materials which can be used to make art programs and facilities more accessible to handicapped people.

Information Services: Publications are available from the Information Service on the following topics: arts for visually impaired persons; arts education for disabled students; making arts programs and facilities accessible to handicapped persons; model programs and facilities; 504 and the visual arts; 504 and the performing arts; funding sources; and sources of technical assistance. In addition, the Service has compiled an annotated bibliography on media for the handicapped, including captioned films and braille arts. A copy of Section 504 regulations is available in large print for visually impaired persons.

A variety of media materials on arts and the handicapped is distributed to interested groups. The collection includes two new slide-tape presentations—*Disabled Artists and Involvement of Disabled People in the Arts* and *Programmatic Accommodations for Arts Institutions.*

Anyone interested in arts and the handicapped may be placed on the Service's mailing list and will receive current materials and information about new editions as they become available. There is no charge for this service.

**National Center for a Barrier Free
    Environment (NCBFE)**
1140 Connecticut Avenue, N.W.
Suite 1006
Washington, DC 20036
(202) 466-6896 (Voice or TTY)

Handicapping Conditions Served: All physical handicaps.

The Organization: The National Center for a Barrier Free Environment (NCBFE) was formed in 1974 as the result of a national conference on barrier free design, where it was recommended that a national organization be established to serve as a central coordinating information collection and disseminating service in support of the barrier free environment movement. The Center's membership includes organizations serving handicapped people, design professionals, rehabilitation professionals, consumer groups, and disabled individuals.

The Center has served as an information clearinghouse, disseminating publications on accessibility issues and responding to technical inquiries relating to accessibility issues. A recent grant from the Community Services Administration and the Office for Civil Rights (HEW) will allow the Center to expand its clearinghouse activities—specifically to computerize its information, and to expand its public information and publications programs. In addition, the Center intends to set up a network of design resource persons in each state who will be available to consult with organizations needing technical assistance.

Information Services: NCBFE provides information to any lay or professional person. The Center collects and disseminates both general and technical information developed by member groups on the removal of architectural barriers. Resource files include information on accessibility standards, codes, projects, programs, equipment, new products, and other relevant technical information. The information will be computerized in the near future, facilitating customized information searches. The Center plans to expand its operation in the area of preparation of resource packets for dealing with specific problems of architectural barriers, such as housing design, kitchen design, etc.

NCBFE publishes technical assistance manuals and booklets which are available at a nominal charge. They include:

1) *Planning for Accessibility*—a manual on developing and implementing campus accessibility transition plans.

2) *Opening Doors*—provides structural planning guidelines on modifications of existing structures.

3) *Accessibility Assistance*—listings of organizations and individuals active in the barrier free design movement.

The Center publishes a bimonthly awareness newsletter, *Report*, which contains information on new publications, conferences, activities, and new developments in the field. Subscriptions are available only to members; single issues are provided free.

National Center for Health Statistics
Health Resources Administration
Public Health Service, HEW
3700 East-West Highway, Room 1-57
Hyattsville, MD 20782
(301) 436-8500

Handicapping Conditions Served: All handicapping conditions.

The Organization: The National Center for Health Statistics (NCHS) is the only federal agency established specifically to collect and disseminate data on health in the United States. The Center designs and maintains national data collection systems, conducts research in statistical and survey methodology, and cooperates with other agencies in the United States and in foreign countries to increase the availability and usefulness of health data.

Through its survey and inventories, the Center produces and disseminates data on illness and disability and on their prevalence and impact in the population. Data have been collected on a number of handicapping conditions; data on the prevalence of most conditions include some indicators of severity and impact. Also collected are data on the supply and use of health services.

Information Services: The primary information service of NCHS is distribution of its statistical data through published reports, which include the following:

Facts at Your Fingertips: A Guide to Sources of Statistical Information on Major Health Topics identifies major areas of interest and describes the kinds of data now available or in preparation. Sources include NCHS publications or data, HEW and other federal offices, and private organizations and associations.

The Vital and Health Statistics Series contains data on program and collection procedures, evaluation and methods research, and analytical studies. This series includes publications on: 1) the Health Interview Survey, which gives statistics on illness, disability, accidental injuries, and the use of hospital, medical, dental, and other services; and 2) the Health Examination Survey, which provides data from direct examination, testing, and measurement of national samples and from which are calculated distributions of the population with respect to physical, physiological, and psychological characteristics.

Advance Data from Vital and Health Statistics is a publication series begun in 1976 as the means for early release of selected findings from the health and demographic surveys of NCHS. Most of these releases are followed by detailed reports in the *Vital and Health Statistics Series.*

The Current Listing and Topical Index to the Vital and Health Statistics Series is an index to the *Vital and Health Statistics Series* and *Advance Data from Vital and Health Statistics* according to demographic and socioeconomic variables. Section 1 includes topics and variables related to the health status of people; Section II covers the characteristics of health facilities and manpower. In addition, titles of published reports are given for each series.

Single copies of most NCHS publications are available free of charge from the Center. Publication orders may be recorded on the 24-hour publications hotline: (301) 436-NCHS. Multiple copies may be obtained from the Superintendent of Documents, U.S. Government Printing Office, Washington, DC 20402. Some titles are out of print at NCHS and may be purchased from the National Technical Information Service (see separate entry). For information on the availability of specific reports, requestors may telephone NCHS at (301) 436-8500.

**Nation Center for Law and the
     Handicapped, Inc. (NCLH)
P.O. Box 477
University of Notre Dame
Notre Dame, IN 46556
(219) 283-4536**

Handicapping Conditions Served: All handicaps.

The Organization: The National Center for Law and the Handicapped was established in 1972 to work for equal protection under the law for all handicapped individuals through provision of legal assistance, legal research activities, and programs of public and professional education and awareness. Although NCLH has served as counsel in court cases, it generally serves in an amicus curiae (friend of the court) role. The legal staff provides assistance to attorneys, protection and advocacy systems, and legislators through consultation, legal research and the drafting of model pleadings and briefs. The Center also provides technical assistance to legal advocacy groups and law school advocacy internship programs.

Information Services: Briefs, monographs and other written materials are available on each of the Center's legal research areas. These areas include: Section 504 of the Rehabilitation Act, deinstitutionalization, zoning and housing, transportation, architectural barriers, employment, education, guardianship, parental rights, ethical issues, and legal protection of the mentally retarded offender. NCLH publishes a bimonthly journal, AMICUS, which reports on the developments in the law as they relate to the rights of the disabled. Each issue focuses on a specific topic, such as the Supreme Court and the handicapped, ethics, advocates in education, and architectural barriers. AMICUS is disseminated to both the lay and legal public.

The Center provides referrals to attorneys with experience representing handicapped persons.

National Center for Research
in Vocational Education
The Ohio State University
1960 Kenny Road
Columbus, OH 43210
(800) 848-4815 (except Ohio)
(614) 486-3655 (Ohio)

Handicapping Conditions Served: All handicaps.

The Organization: The National Center for Research in Vocational Education, established in 1965, is an independent unit of Ohio State University. Approximately half of the Center's funding is provided by the U.S. Office of Education. The main function of the Center is to increase the ability of diverse agencies and organizations to solve educational problems related to career planning, preparation, and progression through: 1) generation of knowledge by means of primary research on career problems and service delivery; 2) development of educational programs and products, which include teachers' guides, staff development modules, and community involvement materials; 3) operation of a variety of information services; and 4) conducting leadership development and training programs.

Information Services: The Center selects a number of vocational education products for national dissemination, some of which focus on the needs of disabled persons (mainstreaming, characteristics of handicapped students, evaluation and placement, architectual considerations, and guidance and counseling services). Materials on various aspects of vocational and career education, including programs for special needs populations, are announced in the *Quarterly Reference List*, available at no charge from the Center.

Another Center periodical, *Resources in Vocational Education*, lists information on research and instructional materials, ongoing research and development projects, and resource organizations. In addition, requestors may obtain copies of an annotated bibliography of research and development projects conducted since 1970, mini-lists of resource organizations in selected areas, and a bibliography of the Center's publications, which number over 700. These publications may be purchased from the Center.

When appropriate, the Center refers inquirers to Center specialists or outside organizations. Persons interested in obtaining bibliographies on specific topics may request custom computer searches at the ERIC Clearinghouse on Adult, Career, and Vocational Education, which is housed at the Center (see ERIC entries). There is no charge for the Center's information service. There is a fee, however, for ERIC searches.

Technical assistance to agencies and organizations is available in many different areas, including needs assessment, research and program planning, and curriculum design. The fee for this service varies according to the type of assistance required.

Requestors interested in purchasing the Center's publications may contact the Publications Office. All inquiries on the Center's programs and activities are handled by the Program Information Office. Both of these offices may be reached at the above telephone numbers.

**National Clearing House of Rehabilitation
   Training Materials**
Oklahoma State University
115 Old USDA Building
Stillwater, OK 74074
(405) 624-7650

Handicapping Conditions Served: All handicapping conditions.

The Organization: The National Clearing House of Rehabilitation Training Materials (NCHRTM), located at Oklahoma State University, is funded by the Rehabilitation Services Administration, Department of Health, Education, and Welfare, to disseminate information on rehabilitation with primary concentration on training materials for use by educators of rehabilitation counselors. Personnel working in the areas of staff development, inservice training, and continuing education are also served by the Clearing House.

NCHRTM houses a collection of "fugitive" materials and information not generally found in traditional libraries. The Clearing House reference collection contains about 3,000 titles in hard copy of microfiche format, back issues of major journals in the rehabilitation field, and various types of audiovisuals. Included in this collection are publications of the Institute on Rehabilitation Issues (formerly the Institute on Rehabilitation Services), which works to identify areas in vocational rehabilitation where training materials are needed and to develop training resources materials in content areas of priority interest with active participation by state vocational rehabilitation personnel. Recent studies in this series focus on rehabilitation engineering, independent living, vocational rehabilitation of severely handicapped persons, and other topics.

Information Services: NCHRTM usually has between 250 and 300 titles to distribute free to requestors in the rehabilitation field. Microfiche or xerox copies of other publications in the Clearing House collection can be made for a cost recovery fee.

An annotated bibliographic newsletter, *NCHRTM Memorandum*, on publications available from the Clearing House and other sources is published quarterly. Materials in rehabilitation and related areas are reviewed as a current awareness service. A bibliography listing Institute on Rehabilitation Issues publications is also available.

NCHRTM helps inquirers identify publications relevant to their information needs, making referrals to outside organizations when necessary. Clearing House services are available primarily to professionals who have training interests in rehabilitation and related fields.

**National Clearinghouse for Alcohol
   Information**
P.O. Box 2345
Rockville, MD 20852
(301) 468-2600

Handicapping Conditions Served: Alcoholism.

The Organization: The Clearinghouse was established in 1972 to make current knowledge on alcohol-related subjects widely available. Part of the National Institute on Alcohol Abuse and Alcoholism, it is operated for the Federal Government by Informatics, Inc. The Clearinghouse has an information program for lay and professional users that includes the dissemination of materials on the prevention, cause, current, and understanding of alcoholism.

Information Services: Reference services and printed materials are available free of charge to any interested individuals. Custom computer searches of the Clearinghouse's data base, which contains more than 40,000 references, may be requested at no charge to the user. Information for practitioners on the administration and operation of an alcoholism program or treatment center is particularly strong.

Medical research is also covered. Public education tools, including radio and television spots and posters, are developed and distributed by the Clearinghouse. Information on alcoholism in persons with mental retardation, epilepsy, hearing impairments, visual impairments, and other handicapping conditions is available.

Users of the Clearinghouse may register for a selected dissemination of information program by completing interest cards. They will then receive monthly listings of additions to the Clearinghouse's data base in their particular areas of interest.

Publications produced by the Clearinghouse include the following: 1) a catalog providing citations to films and other audiovisuals; 2) *Information and Feature Services*, a periodical on trends, opinions and programs across the nation; and 3) *Alcohol Health and Research World*, a quarterly bulletin for researchers and treatment specialists, available from the Superintendent of Documents, U.S. Government Printing Office, Washington, DC 20402. A publication list of other titles available may be requested.

**National Clearinghouse for Drug
   Abuse Information
National Institute of Drug Abuse
Alcohol, Drug Abuse, and Mental Health
   Administration, HEW
5600 Fishers Lane, Room 10-A53
Rockville, MD 20857
(301) 443-6500**

Handicapping Conditions Served: Drug Abuse.

The Organization: Established in 1970 by an act of Congress, the National Clearinghouse for Drug Abuse Information is the central source in the Federal Government for collection and dissemination of information on drug abuse. Part of the National Institute of Drug Abuse (NIDA), it is responsible for providing information on the treatment and prevention of drug abuse, the rehabilitation and maintenance of persons who abuse drugs, psychosocial services available, and research into the drug abuse problem.

Information Services: The Clearinghouse responds to inquiries from researchers, administrators, and other professionals, students, and the general public by disseminating information packets on drugs and their effects, including fact sheets, short reference lists, research monographs and issue papers, and other public education and research literature. Treatment manuals for medical personnel, guides for training drug abuse workers, parent education materials, booklets on minority drug abuse, and information on drug abuse written in Spanish are available. Professionals seeking research information not available at the Clearinghouse are, when appropriate, referred to NIDA researchers.

Requestors may borrow books and films via inter-library loan from the NIDA Resource Center, a library operated by the Clearinghouse containing over 7,500 titles. Photocopies of journal and magazine articles are available directly from the Resource Center. The Clearinghouse also operates the Drug Abuse Communications Network (DRACON), which provides publications and technical assistance to local drug information centers.

There is no charge for Clearinghouse services or publications.

National Clearinghouse for Family
   Planning Information
P.O. Box 2225
Rockville, MD 20852
(301) 881-9400

Handicapping Conditions Served: All handicaps.

The Organization: The National Clearinghouse for Family Planning Information was established in 1976 by the Bureau of Community Health Services, Department of Health, Education, and Welfare, and is operated by Capital Systems, Inc. The Clearinghouse collects and disseminates information on family planning and related topics. Its document collection includes information on contraception, human sexuality, sex education, family planning (both for the general public and for the mentally and physically impaired), and venereal diseases.

Information Services: The Clearinghouse provides materials to clients and staff members in federally supported service agencies and to private sector family planning workers, educators, and consumers. The following services and publications are available, free of charge: 1) subject searches of the Clearinghouse document collection, accessed through an automated retrieval system; 2) bibliographies on special topics, geared to professionals; 3) catalogs of family planning materials; 4) two periodicals—the *Health Education Bulletin*, which provides information on selected health education topics for clinic staff members, and the *Information Services Bulletin*, which lists materials and resources on specific topics; and 5) fact sheets on various aspects of family planning and human sexuality. While none of these publications treats sexuality and disabled persons, the Clearinghouse is able to supply titles and sources of publications in this area.

National Clearinghouse for Human
   Genetic Diseases
1776 East Jefferson Street
Rockville, MD 20852
(301) 279-4642

Handicapping Conditions Served: Genetic diseases.

The Organization: The National Clearinghouse for Human Genetic Diseases was established in October 1978 by the Genetic Services Program, Bureau of Community Health Services, Department of Health, Education, and Welfare. The Clearinghouse collects and disseminates information on the psychological, social, legal, and medical aspects of genetic diseases, which number about 2,800.

Information Services: One of the Clearinghouse's objectives is to assess the need for materials for lay persons and professionals, and recommend the development of resources to meet these needs. A catalog of print and nonprint materials for professional and lay audiences, *Human Genetics: Information and Educational Materials*, issued periodically, is available free of charge. A small but growing collection of books, periodicals and pamphlets is housed in the Clearinghouse library, which may be visited by interested inquirers.

The Clearinghouse has developed an in-house computerized data base containing information on genetic resources and services, which is searched by the staff in order to retrieve listings of publications, organizations, programs, and legislation to meet individual requests. The Clearinghouse also has access to the Birth Defects Information System, a joint project of the March of Dimes Birth Defects Foundation, Tufts University, and the Massachusetts Institute of Technology. This automated system provides information on genetic diseases including recent findings, treatment, prognosis, complications, and bibliographic references (described under entry March of Dimes Birth Defects Foundation).

A national listing of clinical genetic services centers, indexed by state and city, is available from the Clearinghouse. In addition, the Clearinghouse staff provides technical assistance to organizations which are involved in the development of educational materials. Services of the Clearinghouse are available at no charge to primary health care providers (clinicians, social workers, nurses, etc.), patients, family members of patients, and the general public.

**National Clearinghouse for Mental
    Health Information
National Institute of Mental Health,
    HEW
11A-33 Parklawn Building
5600 Fishers Lane
Rockville, MD 20857
(301) 443-4513 for inquiries and publications
(301) 443-4517 for computer services**

Handicapping Conditions Served: Mental and emotional disorders.

The Organization: The National Clearinghouse for Mental Health Information was established in 1963 in response to the need for centralizing all sources of mental health information, and is responsible for the collection, storage, retrieval, and dissemination of scientific information in the area of mental health. The Clearinghouse collects and abstracts the world's mental health literature. This information, classified and stored in a bibliographic data base, includes data on journals, books, films, technical reports, monographs, and workshop and conference proceedings for many countries and in many languages.

Information Services: Custom searches of the Clearinghouse's data base are available upon request to professionals, and yield bibliographies and abstracts of mental health literature and lists of audiovisual materials tailored to meet specific inquiries. Searches usually include current material (over 65,000 items from the past two or three years). Retrospective searches of records from 1963 (over 300,000 citations) may be arranged if warranted by the user's need for information. The NIMH data base (1969 to present) may also be accessed through Bibliographic Retrieval Services (see Data Base Vendors, page 97).

Exhibit and film information on mental health is also available. Except for subscription publications which must be ordered from the Superindendent of Documents, U.S. Government Printing Office, Washington, DC 20402, single copies of Clearinghouse publications may be obtained from the Clearinghouse without charge.

When appropriate, requestors are referred to other agencies and organizations. Individuals seeking treatment are referred to community mental health centers and state hospitals.

**National Clearinghouse on Aging
Administration on Aging, HEW
330 Independence Avenue, S.W.
Washington, DC 20201
(202) 245-2158**

Handicapping Conditions Served: All handicaps, although information is limited to aging persons (age 60 and over).

The Organization: The Administration on Aging (AOA) is the principal federal agency concerned with identifying the needs, concerns, and interests of older persons and with the administration of the programs of the Older Americans Act. AOA is also the principal agency for promoting coordination of federal resources available to meet the needs of older persons.

The goal of the National Clearinghouse on Aging is to collect, analyze, and disseminate information on the problems and circumstances of the aging population and their impact on the social system. The wide range of subject areas covered by the Clearinghouse includes nutrition, housing, health, employment, supportive social services, legislation, and training for professionals who work with aging persons.

Information Services: The Clearinghouse responds to inquiries on all aspects of aging by sending copies of Clearinghouse fact sheets, bibliographies, and other publications. When appropriate, inquirers are referred to other information centers or to direct service providers, including the state agencies on aging, which offer a variety of services to older Americans. Fact sheets are available on federal programs which assist the elderly, employment and volunteer opportunities for older persons, educational possibilities for older persons, retirement housing, crime prevention, transportation, recreation, audiovisual materials sponsored by AoA, and other topics. A brochure entitled *To Find the Way* outlines major sources of assistance for older Americans.

The Clearinghouse also compiles statistical information on the aging population, summarized in a pamphlet, *Facts About Older Americans. Statistical Reports on Older Americans, Number 3,* one of the series of publications giving more detailed data, describes the most recent Census Bureau projections of the elderly population to the year 2035, and discusses some of the implications for such characteristics as health, income, living arrangements, and other variables. The *Cumulative Index of AoA Discretionary Grants and Contracts,* issued approximately once a year, lists all projects funded by AoA. There is no charge for these publications.

SCAN, the Service Center for Aging Information, is the component of the Clearinghouse which sponsors a bibliographic information retrieval system under contract. The system consists of a Central Control Facility for processing documents and three Resource Centers for collecting, indexing, and abstracting documents.

Two of the Resource Centers are now available to answer inquiries in specialized areas: 1) social practice: Service Center for Aging Information, Social Practice Resource Center, P.O. Box 168, Silver Spring, Maryland 20907 (800/638-2051); and 2) social and behavioral sciences: Service Center for Aging Information, Social-Behavioral Sciences Resource Center, P.O. Box 15943, Philadelphia, Pennsylvania 19103 (800/523-0793). Upon request, these centers will provide bibliographies on any topic in their respective fields. The SCAN system will also provide microfiche or paper copies of many of the documents listed on the bibliographies for a fee.

National Diabetes Information
    Clearinghouse
805 15th St., N.W.
Suite 500
Washington, DC 20005
(202) 638-7620

Handicapping Conditions Served: Diabetes.

The Organization: The Clearinghouse is a service of the National Institute of Arthritis, Metabolism, and Digestive Diseases (NIADD) and is designed to speed the exchange of information among all private and public groups engaged in diabetes educational programs for professionals, patients, and the public. The Clearinghouse also initiates the preparation of new materials and sponsors workshops and conferences for the exchange of current scientific information. Primary users are health care professionals.

Information Services: The Clearinghouse distributes information to health care professionals about materials available elsewhere. For the lay inquirer, very general information and referral to other organizations is available, including referral to state or regional health agencies and to the major voluntary diabetes organizations. Clearinghouse publications are primarily topical annotated bibliographies and a newsletter, *Diabetes Dateline*, which covers programs, news items, and materials available from various sources. Bibliographies of professional and patient materials span the many aspects and subjects related to diabetes: foot care; diet and nutrition; the visually impaired diabetic; the adult with limited reading skills; children and youth; career and employment information for diabetics; diabetic aids; psychosocial and behavioral studies; a resource list of programs and projects; and many others.

National Eye Institute (NEI)
National Institutes of Health, HEW
Building 31, Room 6A25
Bethesda, MD 20205
(301) 496-5248

Handicapping Conditions Served: Blindness and visual impairments.

The Organization: The National Eye Institute (NEI) has primary responsibility within the National Institutes of Health and the Federal Government for supporting and conducting research aimed at improving prevention, diagnosis and treatment of visual disorders. In addition, NEI encourages the application of research findings to clinical practice, heightens public awareness of vision problems, and cooperates with voluntary organizations which engage in related activities.

Information Services: Printed material on the following eye conditions is available upon request: cataract, retinal detachment, glaucoma, refractive errors, corneal diseases, macular degeneration, diabetic retinopathy, and retinitis pigmentosa. Also available are statistics on eye disease and visual impairment, and information on NEI-supported research. In addition, NEI can refer people to other information sources and refer inquiries regarding assistance for people with eye disorders or visual impairments to the appropriate agency, organization, or health provider.

National Health Information
    Clearinghouse (NHIC)
1550 Wilson Boulevard
Suite 600
Rosslyn, VA 22209
(703) 522-2590

Handicapping Conditions Served: All handicaps.

The Organization: Scheduled to become operational in the late spring of 1980, the National Health Information Clearinghouse (NHIC) is a project of the Office of Health Information, Health Promotion, and Physical Fitness and Sports Medicine (OHIHP), of the U.S. Department of Health, Education, and Welfare. In addition to its clearinghouse function, NHIC will initiate liaison activities in order to encourage the exchange of ideas on common concerns and goals among health information providers.

Information Services: NHIC will operate as a referral center. Its data base of resource organizations will help consumers find the health information they need by locating the appropriate sources of the information. It is expected that source information will be entered into a computerized file, allowing on-line access to the data. Resource organizations will include disease prevention and health promotion programs, clearinghouses, libraries, hospitals, educational institutions, voluntary organizations, and government agencies at the local, state, national, and international levels. Organizations which provide information on the following topics will be included: nutrition, cancer, immunization, accident control, infectious diseases, acupuncture, fluoridation, teenage pregnancy, hypertension, smoking, biofeedback, self care, risk assessment, and physical fitness.

It is expected that NHIC's referral services will be available free of charge to lay persons and professionals. Brochures and bibliographies on topics of current interest and a monthly newsletter will be published. There may be a charge for some publications.

National Heart, Lung, and Blood
   Institute (NHLBI)
National Institutes of Health, HEW
Building 31, Room 4A21
Bethesda, MD 20205
(301) 496-4236

Handicapping Conditions Served: Cardiovascular disorders, respiratory conditions including black lung disease, stroke, and blood disorders (including hemophilia, Cooley's anemia, and sickle cell disease).

The Organization: NHLBI funds a multimillion dollar research program at its own headquarters and around the country at universities and medical schools. Research and professional training are done on diseases of the heart, blood vessels, blood and lung, and in the use of blood and the management of blood resources.

Information Services: The focus of the Institute's information services is the **Public Inquiries and Reports Branch**. All information activities are aimed at reducing illness and death from heart, lung, and blood diseases. Advances in research are translated through press conferences, pamphlets, fact sheets, exhibits for use by professionals and lay audiences, audiovisuals, and special projects. Conference proceedings for scientists are prepared regularly, and professional and public education materials are made widely available.

Anyone may request information and most is provided free. Fees are levied for bibliographies, indexes or abstracts that must be specially prepared. On-site use of NHLBI holdings of books, indexes, journals, or search and retrieval systems is permitted. Numerous professional and general publications are available. A list of current publications and materials produced by NHLBI shows dozens of resources which can be ordered.

Dietary and nutrition information is in abundance at the Institute. Nutrition games have been developed for distribution through local chapters of the American Heart Association. A dietary series for patients with lipid disorders has been distributed throughout the world, accompanied by a companion handbook for physicians.

Audiovisuals available on loan include exhibits on cardiopulmonary resuscitation, diabetes, and cardiovascular disease, high blood pressure, "food for thought," and sickle cell disease. A film, "Alive Today," covers heart disease and research advances and is available from the American Heart Association.

A series of seminars for biology teachers on how to teach about sickle cell disease includes slides, filmstrips, and tests.

NHLBI also supports **National Research and Demonstration Centers** and clinical studies throughout the country, which generate their own materials and are a community source of information. For example, a center at the University of Vermont expedites translation of research findings on lung diseases into practical patient care in local communities; the center also coordinates the activities of several state and local groups concerned with respiratory diseases.

A task force on respiratory diseases has issued a report that will serve as the basic research plan for NHLBI for the next ten years. Several educational programs are being planned on various lung diseases, as a result of the task force work.

National detection, prevention and control programs are conducted for high blood pressure and sickle cell disease.

The **National High Blood Pressure Education Program** coordinates the work of more than 150 private, Federal, voluntary, and professional organizations in preventing and controlling the disorder, and in educating professionals and the public about the problem. Information activities are centered in the national **High Blood Pressure Information Center** (see separate entry), which answers public inquiries and distributes free educational materials and reprints from professional and lay periodicals.

Through the **Sickle Cell Disease Program**, NHLBI has established a number of Sickle Cell Screening and

Education Clinics and Comprehensive Sickle Cell Centers throughout the country. Various educational and public awareness activities are supported by these centers.

**National Information Center for Special
    Education Materials (NICSEM)
University of Southern California
University Park
Los Angeles, CA 90007
(800) 421-8711 (except California)
(213) 741-5899 (California residents may call collect)**

Handicapping Conditions Served: All handicapping conditions.

The Organization: Funded by the Bureau of Education for the Handicapped, Department of Health, Education, and Welfare, the National Information Center for Special Education Materials (NICSEM) is a computerized bibliographic information retrieval system containing more than 36,000 records of commercially available audiovisuals, print and braille materials, equipment, and adaptive devices for all educational levels of handicapped persons, although most materials are for use with children. NICSEM indexes materials applicable to all types of handicapping conditions, including materials in the following areas: cognition and perception, motor processes, career and vocational education, guidance, language, instructional approaches, minority groups, and specific subjects such as mathematics and science.

Established in 1977, NICSEM has been able to draw on the resources of the **National Information Center for Educational Media (NICEM)**, also located at the University of Southern California.

Information Services: NICSEM plans to publish a variety of indexes produced from the NICSEM data base, including the *Parent Index*, now available, which includes materials for use by parents with children and professional materials for use by teachers and administrators in providing guidance or training to parents. A master index of the complete data base, indexes to assessment and in-service training materials, and mini-indexes in several areas will be published in 1980. NICSEM indexes will allow professionals to identify appropriate materials based on the instructional objectives contained in the student's Individual Education Program.

Because the NICEM data base, which is limited to audiovisuals, was found to contain a wealth of information on special education, for the most part not duplicating records in the NICSEM file, NICEM and NICSEM have collaborated in the publication of the NICEM *Index to Nonprint Special Education Materials–Multimedia* which comes in two sections: 1) "Learner Volume," which contains over 35,000 titles and abstracts on materials suitable for direct instruction of the handicapped; and 2) "Professional Volume," which contains over 5,000 abstracts of materials for use by parents, teachers, and other professionals. Both of these indexes are available from NICSEM in paper and microfiche formats.

There is a charge for indexes and for most other NICSEM publications, which include the *Thesaurus*, of interest to those who wish to conduct searches of the data base. Computer searches of the NICSEM data base are available from Bibliographic Retrieval Services and Lockheed (see Data Base Vendors, page 97).

**National Institute of Allergy and
    Infectious Diseases (NIAID)
National Institute of Health, HEW
Building 31, Room 7A32
Bethesda, MD 20205
(301) 496-5717**

Handicapping Conditions Served: Allergies and infectious diseases of all kinds; also transplantation and immune deficiency disease. The focus is on acute infections, and on the conditions that lead to chronic diseases affecting the handicapped.

The Organization: NIAID supports a multimillion dollar research effort across the country at research institutions, aimed at a better understanding of the causes of allergic, immunologic, and infectious diseases and to the development of better means of preventing, diagnosing, and healing these illnesses. Some of the studies are of infectious agents found in other countries, which cause death or severe handicaps for people living in the tropics and other areas outside of the U.S. (e.g., malaria and other parasitic diseases, leprosy, cholera, and viral diarrheas).

NIAID supports **Asthma and Allergic Disease Centers** in 15 institutions which translate basic concepts in immunology, genetics, biochemistry and pharmacology into clinical research. Four **Comprehensive Immunologic Research and Disease Centers** study immunologic diseases.

Information Services: NIAID provides general information about disorders currently being studied at the Asthma and Allergic Disease Centers and the Immunologic Centers. A 10-minute slide show is available on "What You Should Know about Asthma." Coming soon is another slide presentation on "How to Cope with Your Environment If You Have Allergies." The Institute has numerous publications for the lay person which cover the range of infectious diseases and allergies (e.g., asthma, sarcoidosis, systemic fungal diseases, sinusitis, the common cold, influenza, viral hepatitis, strep infections). Booklets are also available on viruses and bacteria and on hospital associated infections, pneumococcal infections, sexually transmitted diseases, and antiviral substances.

NIAID does not make referrals to sources of financial assistance for medical care, transportation, etc.

**National Institute of Arthritis, Metabolism
and Digestive Diseases (NIAMDD)
National Institutes of Health, HEW
Building 31, Room 9A04
Bethesda, MD 20205
(301) 496-3583**

Handicapping Conditions Served: Arthritis, diabetes, digestive diseases, endocrine and metabolic disorders, kidney and urinary tract infections. Specific disorders include such diseases as: ulcer, colitis, ileitis, systemic lupus erythematosus, gout, scoliosis, cystic fibrosis, osteogenesis imperfecta, and others.

The Organization: NIAMDD supports millions of dollars of research each year on the causes of and improved treatment for more than 100 different forms of tissue diseases; diabetes and other metabolic disorders; digestive diseases and nutrition; diseases of the kidney and urinary tract; and certain diseases of the bones and skin. NIAMDD also supports **Multipurpose Arthritis Centers** that emphasize research and pilot programs in health education. Most centers have clinics.

Information Services: NIAMDD's **Arthritis Information Clearinghouse** and its **National Diabetes Information Clearinghouse** (see separate entries) work with health educators and health professionals and handle requests for professional literature. At the central information office of NIAMDD (address above), basic brochures are available on *How to Cope with Arthritis, How to Cope with Diabetes,* and on several other subjects (cystic fibrosis, scoliosis, kidney dialysis, systemic lupus erythematosus, peptic ulcer, and gout). Most information is in printed form. A list of the NIAMDD **Multipurpose Arthritis Centers** is also available.

**National Institute of Child Health
and Human Development (NICHD)**
National Institutes of Health, HEW
Building 31, Room 2A34
Bethesda, MD 20205
(301) 496-5133

Handicapping Conditions Served: Mental retardation (particularly Down's syndrome) and learning disabilities (particularly dyslexia). A few genetic and metabolic disorders are studied.

The Organization: NICHD funds a multimillion dollar research program at its headquarters and around the country, at universities and medical schools. Research and doctoral training are done in the areas of maternal and child health, human development, and reproduction/population, with the focus on the continuing growth and development process (biological and behavioral) from the prenatal period to maturity. The NICHD also supports 12 **Mental Retardation Research Centers** across the country, where research, professional education, patient care, and counseling are undertaken.

Information Services: Information is particularly strong on research related to Down's syndrome, mental retardation, speech and language, and speech and reading. Most information describes various conditions and what is currently known about them. Patients may be referred by NICHD to the programs of the **Mental Retardation Research Centers** for diagnosis, treatment, and other services. Publications for the public include *Developmental Dyslexia and Related Reading Disorders*, and other speech/reading and speech/language materials; and booklets on Down's syndrome, low birth weight babies, and sudden infant death. For the professional, materials cover antenatal diagnosis and amniocentesis, adolescent sexuality, smoking during pregnancy and adolescence, and other topics.

National Institute of Dental Research (NIDR)
National Institutes of Health, HEW
Building 31, Room 2C34
Bethesda, MD 20205
(301) 496-4261

Handicapping Conditions Served: Dental diseases and disorders of the craniofacial area, including cleft lip and cleft palate.

The Organization: The National Institute of Dental Research (NIDR) is the chief sponsor of dental research and related postdoctoral training in the United States. NIDR studies relate to the cause, prevention and methods of diagnosis and treatment of dental disease and conditions.

Information Services: The NIDR information program provides members of the specific community, the dental profession and the lay public with reports of dental research progress.

For the professional, periodic issuances of *NIDR Research News* and *Abstracts from NIDR Scientists* provide reports of current research activities and summaries of published research reports. The Institute also funds state-of-the-art conferences and workshops and makes the published proceedings of these meetings available. Exhibits depicting research findings and known methods of dental disease prevention are developed and shown at medical/dental, scientific, and health educator meetings. Films on topical fluorides and dental sealants, both useful methods in the prevention of dental caries in the general public and in the handicapped patient, are available as teaching tools for dental clinicians.

For the layperson, pamphlets on general dental health and on specific health problems of relevance to the Institute (e.g., *Cleft Lip and Cleft Palate*) are distributed to the general public. Inquiries from the public are answered with information from the latest research reports, citations to the general dental literature, and where appropriate, information is supplied regarding grantee institutions where possible service can be offered the handicapped patient.

**National Institute of Neurological
 and Communicative Disorders and Stroke
 (NINCDS)**
National Institutes of Health, HEW
Building 31, Room 8A-06
Bethesda, MD 20205
(301) 496-5751

Handicapping Conditions Served: Neurological disorders in general, communicative disorders in general, cerebrovascular disease, metabolic disorders affecting the nervous system, head and spinal cord injury.

The Organization: NINCDS is one of eleven research institutes making up the National Institutes of Health. The Institute's mission is to conduct, support, and coordinate research in the causes, prevention, diagnosis, and treatment of neurological and communicative disorders and stroke, and in basic sciences relevant to these problems. Support of postdoctoral training for research careers is also a basic component of the Institute's mission.

The Institute supports clinical research centers at university medical complexes, where patient research is conducted on epilepsy, stroke, spinal cord injury, multiple sclerosis, neural prostheses, and other neurological conditions. The Institute also collects and disseminates information on research in its field.

Information Services: NINCDS maintains an Office of Scientific and Health Reports (OSHR) whose services are available free to both lay and professional users. Inquiries about the Institute program, neurological and communicative disorders, and research progress in these fields are answered by phone and mail. Approximately 60 publications are kept in stock and sent out in response to inquiries. Publications include a "Hope through Research" series of 17 pamphlets (many covering disabling conditions), a fact sheet series consisting of 11 titles, and about 10 miscellaneous pamphlets, reprints, and other publications. Annual special reports on research progress in the major neurological and communicative areas are available, as well as scientific and technical documents, such as a monograph series containing reviews, reports of advisory committees, and proceedings of scientific meetings. A publications list and single copies of NINCDS publications are available free to individuals, and organizations may order small quantities for their own distribution.

NINCDS supports scientific reference services in the fields of epilepsy, basic neurosciences, and clinical neurosciences to serve physicians. For bulletins on basic neuroscience topics, contact the Brain Information Service (see separate entry). For bulletins on clinical neurology topics, contact:

Clinical Neurology Information Center
University of Nebraska Medical Center
42nd and Dewey Avenue
Omaha, NE 68105
(402) 541-4925

A monthly news service, "NINCDS Notes," is available to journals and newspapers.

For further information, call or write the Office of Scientific and Health Reports at the above address.

National Library of Medicine (HLM)
National Institutes of Health, HEW
8600 Rockville Pike
Bethesda, MD 20209
(301) 496-6095

Handicapping Conditions Served: All handicaps.

The Organization: The National Library of Medicine is a part of the National Institutes of Health (NIH), one of the six health agencies of the Public Health Service. The Library was established in 1836 as the

Library of the Army Surgeon General's Office and remained under the armed forces until 1956, when it was designated as the National Library of Medicine and placed within the Public Health Service by an act of Congress.

The world's largest research library in a single scientific and professional field, the Library serves as the nation's chief medical information source. The Library, which collects materials exhaustively in approximately 40 biomedical areas, has holdings of about two and a half million books, journals, technical reports, theses, microfilms, and other materials.

Information Services: The Library's computer-based Medical Analysis and Retrieval System (MEDLARS) was established to achieve rapid bibliographic access to NLM's store of biomedical information. It became operational in 1964 with the publication of the first computer-produced issue of *Index Medicus*, a comprehensive, monthly subject-author index to articles from approximately 2,200 of the world's biomedical journals. The principal objective of MEDLARS is to provide references to the biomedical literature for research scientists, clinicians, and other health professionals. MEDLARS contains over four million references dating from 1964 and covering virtually all handicapping conditions, rehabilitation medicine, and rehabilitation engineering. MEDLINE (MEDLARS ON-Line), which became operational in late 1971, provides the capability in medical libraries around the country to query the NLM computer's store of journal article references for quick retrieval. MEDLINE contains over 500,000 recent references.

Other computerized data bases developed by NLM include the following (numbers of records contained in these files are from the summer of 1979):

• *TOXLINE* (Toxicology Information On-Line) is a collection of 520,000 references from the last five years on published human and animal toxicity studies, effects of environmental chemicals, and adverse drug reactions.

• *CANCERLIT* (Cancer Literature) is sponsored by NIH's National Cancer Institute and contains more than 140,000 references on various aspects of cancer.

• *EPILEPSYLINE* is sponsored by NIH's National Institute of Neurological and Communicative Disorders and Stroke. This file contains about 25,000 references and abstracts to articles on epilepsy that have been compiled by Excerpta Medica (see separate entry).

• *AVLINE* (Audiovisuals On-Line) is a file of about 6,000 audiovisual teaching packages used in health sciences education at the college level and for the continuing education of practitioners.

• *HEALTH PLANNING & ADMIN* (Health Planning and Administration) contains about 100,000 references to literature on health planning, organization, financing, management manpower, and related subjects.

• *BIOETHICSLINE*, developed at the Center for Bioethics, Kennedy Institute of Ethics, Georgetown University, gives bibliographic information on questions of ethics and public policy arising in health care or biomedical research. It contains about 6,500 records.

Eleven Regional Medical Libraries, each responsible for a geographic area, coordinate NLM's on-line search services in the U.S. In addition to conducting searches themselves, they can provide the user with the location of the nearest on-line center with access to NLM data bases. (There are over one thousand of these centers located in hospitals, universities, state libraries, organizations, and companies throughout the country.) The charge for NLM searches varies with each Regional Medical Library and local center; in some cases there is no cost to certain classes of users. The Regional Medical Libraries also handle requests for health literature not available locally, referring to NLM requests they cannot fill. Inquirers may contact NLM for the location of the Regional Medical Library serving their area.

NLM publications include *Index Medicus*, described above; bibliographies on drug interactions, toxicity, epidemiology, environmental pollution as related to health, and other subjects; and published literature searches on a variety of topics. A list of publications with ordering information is available upon request.

Direct access to MEDLARS and MEDLINE is also available through Bibliographic Retrieval Services (see Data Base Vendors, page 97).

**National Library Services for the Blind
   and Physically Handicapped**
Library of Congress
1291 Taylor Street, N.W.
Washington, DC 20542
(202) 287-5100

Handicapping Conditions Served: Blindness, visual impairment, deaf/blindness, reading disabilities resulting from organic dysfunction, and any other physical limitation that prevents the normal use of standard printed material.

The Organization: The National Library Service for the Blind and Physically Handicapped (NLS) collection of full-length braille and talking books and magazines produced for blind and physically handicapped readers is loaned free to individuals who cannot hold, handle, or read conventional printed matter. Books, magazines, and playback equipment provided by NLS are distributed through a national network of 160 locally funded cooperating libraries and agencies where they are circulated to eligible residents of the United States and its territories. NLS has developed a national automated bibliographic service that enables cooperating network libraries to identify and locate books produced in special formats for handicapped readers.

NLS trains and certifies volunteers in braille transcribing and in braille proofreading. Eligible readers can request that a local volunteer group braille or record materials they cannot locate elsewhere. *Volunteers Who Produce Books: Braille, Tape, Large Type* is a directory that lists by state the names of volunteer groups and individuals who transcribe and record books and other reading materials for blind and physically handicapped persons. Voice auditions and informal training are given to volunteer tape narrators. The Telephone Pioneers of America, senior or retired telephone industry workers, maintain and repair playback equipment.

Information Services: The national book collection includes more than 25,000 titles of bestsellers, classics, gothic and romantic novels, mysteries, science fiction, history, biography, religion, poetry, essays, how-to-do-it books, foreign language materials, and children's books. The children's collection includes a number of special books that combine print with braille, enabling blind and sighted children and adults to read together. Some of these Print/Braille books are illustrated with fragrance strips that emit scents when scratched. Currently recorded and brailled books are announced in the bimonthly magazines *Talking Book Topics* and *Braille Book Review*. Eligible readers receive these publications in large type, recorded, and/or braille versions.

Seventy magazines on disc, cassette, and in braille are offered through the program. Readers may request free subscriptions to *Harper's, U.S. News and World Report, National Geographic, Sports Illustrated,* and many other popular magazines. Current issues are mailed to readers at about the same time the printed issues appear.

Playback equipment is loaned free to readers for as long as library materials are being borrowed. Talking-book machines are designed to play disc recorded books and magazines at 8 rpm and 16 rpm; cassette book machines are designed for cassettes recorded at 15/16 ips and the standard speed of 1-7/8 ips as well as on 2 tracks and 4 tracks. Available accessories for playback equipment include earphones and pillowphones. An auxiliary amplifier for hearing-impaired persons is available from NLS on special request.

The **NLS Reference Section** provides information on various aspects of blindness and physical handicaps. Requests may be sent to NLS or to any cooperating network library. The service is available without charge to individuals, organizations, and libraries. The NLS reference collection consists of approximately 4,000 print books and 500 professional journals dealing with handicaps and related subjects. The Section maintains extensive vertical files which contain commercial and organizational catalogs, brochures, and newsletters; pamphlets; newsclippings; and other material relating to blindness and physical handicaps. Referral services are made to additional sources, organizations, and agencies.

The Section receives about 20,000 inquiries a year about such topics as recreation, education, and vocations for handicapped individuals; aids and appliances for blind persons; and federal benefits and laws relating to handicapped persons. To answer frequently recurring questions, the Section supplies special reference circulars, bibliographies and information packages. Topics for reference circulars and bibliographies include sources of spoken word recordings; magazines in special media; large type; reading and writing aids for the handicapped; information for handicapped travelers, games and sports for disabled persons; accessibility; braille instruction and writing materials; library services for handicapped individuals; reading machines for the blind; and closed circuit reading devices for the visually impaired. Information package topics include blindness; braile; learning disabilities; service to handicapped students in academic libraries; general compliance with sections 503 and 504 of the Rehabilitation Act of 1973; information for teachers or for parents of handicapped children; and information for teachers and parents about blind children.

The **NLS Music Section** provides music materials directly to musicians and music students. The collection consists of 30,000 music books and periodicals in braille, large-print, and recorded formats; braille and large type music scores; and instructional cassettes. The music staff performs bibliographic searches for materials, answers brief informational questions, and refers patrons to volunteers who produce braille, recorded, or large-print music transcriptions of specifically requested materials that have not been produced.

Blind and physically handicapped persons who wish to borrow materials may contact NLS for the location of the nearest cooperating library. Eligible U.S. citizens living abroad and music patrons are served directly from NLS. Reading materials are sent to borrowers and returned to libraries by postage-free mail.

**National Rehabilitation Information
    Center (NARIC)**
4407 Eighth Street, N.E.
The Catholic University of America
Washington, DC 20064
(202) 635-5822 (Voice)
(202) 635-5885 (TTY)

Handicapping Conditions Served: All handicaps.

The Organization: The National Rehabilitation Information Center (NARIC) is a rehabilitation research library funded by the National Institute of Handicapped Research (NIHR), Department of Health, Education, and Welfare, to improve the delivery of information to the rehabilitation community. NARIC's collection includes documents and audiovisual materials relevant to the rehabilitation of all disability groups, as well as materials on professional and administrative practices and concerns. The NARIC computerized data base, which covers all aspects of the rehabilitation field, contains bibliographic data and abstracts on reports and audiovisuals in the Center's collection.

NARIC works closely with other information providers through an informal network for the exchange of information on current rehabilitation issues, needs, and information activities.

Information Services: NARIC performs customized searches of its bibliographic data base and of other relevant commercially available computerized data bases. There is a charge for these services. Copies of documents may be obtained for a nominal photocopying fee. The "NARIC Thesaurus," used to index rehabilitation materials, and the bimonthly newsletter, *Pathfinder*, may also be purchased. Braille editions are available. Prepared bibliographies listing publications and audiovisuals on topics of high interest are available at no charge. Among subjects covered are architectural and attitudinal barriers, daily living, deinstitutionalization, homebound persons, independent living, recreation, transportation, and work evaluation.

NARIC's information specialists provide reference services, helping inquirers locate names, addresses, statistics, and other factual information. Users may consult NARIC's collection of books and audiovisuals at the Center. A list of journals and newsletters housed in the library is available free of charge; publishers' names and addresses are included. NARIC's computerized data base will be available through Bibliographic Retrieval Services in mid-1980 (see Data Base Vendors, page 97).

National Technical Information Service
U.S. Department of Commerce
5285 Port Royal Road
Springfield, VA 22161
(703) 557-4600 (for general information)
(703) 557-4642 (to order search)
(703) 557-4650 (to order documents)

Handicapping Conditions Served: All handicaps.

The Organization: The National Technical Information Service (NTIS) is an agency created by Congress in 1950 to provide technical reports and other information products of specialized interest to business, educators, government, and the public. NTIS is the central source for the public sale of U.S. and foreign government sponsored research, development and engineering reports, and other analyses prepared by national and local government agencies, their contractors or grantees, and other technical groups. The NTIS information collection exceeds one million titles, all for purchase. About 150,000 of these are foreign origin. As directed under legislative mandate, NTIS functions on a cost recovery basis; all the cost of its products and services are paid from sales income.

Information Services: Customers may use NTIS's on-line computer search service to identify abstracts of interest from the Bibliographic Data File, which contains 750,000 federally sponsored research reports completed and published from 1964 to date. Most of the documents cited are available only through NTIS. This data base contains documents on handicapping conditions and programs for disabled persons, including rehabilitation, rehabilitation engineering, transportation, and health care. Before initiating a search, users may consult with NTIS information specialists, who will determine the likelihood of retrieval of relevant documents. Published searches on over 1200 topics of wide interest may be ordered from NTIS. These are listed in *Current Published Searches from the NTIS Bibliographic Data File*, available without charge.

The Government Reports Announcements and Index lists summaries of U.S. government research on a bi-weekly basis. It is indexed by subject, personal and cooperate author, and government contract and report numbers. In addition, 26 abstract newsletters provide readers with research summaries within three weeks of their receipt by NTIS from the originating agencies. Abstract newsletters of interest to professionals in the handicapped field include the following: *Behavior and Society, Biomedical Technology and Human Factor Engineering, Health Planning,* and *Medicine and Biology*.

Selected Research in Microfiche (SRIM), a subscription service available in 500 subject categories, provides on a biweekly basis full text microfiche copies of reports in only the subject areas selected by the requestor.

The Federal Software Exchange Center, operated by NTIS, serves as a clearinghouse of federally created computer programs and data files. An annual catalog lists products and the agencies from which they are available.

NTIS publishes many other periodicals and catalogs containing technical information on safety statistics, human services, municipal information systems, and other specialized subjects. In addition, a number of periodicals and reports make available information on research performed outside of the U.S., political and economic analyses of foreign countries, and foreign news releases and articles from periodicals. The free catalog *NTIS Information Services* describes all products and services of the agency.

Direct on-line access to the Bibliographic Data File may be arranged through Bibliographic Retrieval Services, Lockheed, or the System Development Corporation (see Data Base Vendors, page 97).

Office of Cancer Communications
National Cancer Institute (NCI)
National Institutes of Health, HEW
Bethesda, MD 20205
(800) 638-6694
In Maryland: (800) 492-6600
In Alaska and Hawaii: (800) 638-6070

Handicapping Conditions Served: All cancers.

The Organization: NCI conducts and funds the nation's major cancer research program. NCI grants and contracts support cancer research in most of the nation's university medical centers and many other non-Federal institutions. NCI also coordinates the cancer research programs of Federal and private institutions in accordance with a constantly updated National Cancer Plan, which encompasses the lines of research effort considered to be most important in solving the major problems of cancer.

A network of 21 **Comprehensive Cancer Centers** around the country engage in the wide range of cancer related research and demonstration, encompassing basic research, diagnosis, treatment, rehabilitation, public and patient education. The Centers also educate and train professionals in the various clinical and research specialties.

At the community level, patients may be admitted to clinical studies at NCI's **Clinical Cooperative Groups**. Care is paid for by third party assistance or by NCI. These groups exist at 455 institutions, involving 4600 doctors. Drugs are provided free.

NCI also supports 29 **Clinical Cancer Centers**, small centers specializing in cancer treatment.

Information Services: To speed the translation of research results into widespread application, the National Cancer Act of 1971 authorized a **Cancer Control Program** to demonstrate and communicate to both the medical community and general public the latest advances in cancer prevention and management. The program identifies cancer knowledge and technology and makes it available to health practitioners and the public through cooperative efforts with private and community organizations. Prevention, detection, and treatment information is prepared by NCI and distributed through community-based and Comprehensive Cancer Centers' communications offices to high risk groups.

The **Cancer Information Service (CIS)** is a toll-free telephone inquiry system which supplies information about cancer and resources available to cancer patients. CIS offices are in 19 locations associated with the Comprehensive Cancer Centers. About 70 percent of the U.S. population is within the areas directly served by regional CIS offices, and the remainder is served by the CIS at the National Cancer Institute in Bethesda, MD. CIS offices can provide specific information on particular cancer sites, detection programs, local resources for cancer patients (e.g., treatment and rehabilitation facilities, home care assistance, availability of transportation) and facts about the process of patient referral to physicians and consultation among health professionals. Information about possible causes of cancer, how to help prevent cancer, and how different forms of cancer are detected is also available. For the nearest CIS office, consult the white pages of your telephone directory or call the appropriate telephone number listed above.

Patient materials are a strength of the NCI program and many are distributed by physicians. Twenty-five pamphlets on various sites of cancers in the body have been distributed to 45,000 physicians.

NCI's **Organized Dissemination Projects**, multimedia information activities, center on specific topics. Health planners and communicators review the state of knowledge in particular subject areas and a *Digest* of basic information is produced. The *Digest* covers such topics as treatment options, diagnosis, and prevention. Dissemination projects have included smoking, breast cancer, coping with cancer, and asbestos cancer. Hundreds of thousands of patient information and physician kits are distributed, along with posters, slide-tape presentations and booklets on each topic. Materials aimed at motivating patients or high risk groups to take some health action are tested by NCI for effectiveness before being used in the projects.

NCI also supports the **Cancer Information Clearinghouse** (see separate entry), which documents the availability of cancer education materials around the country.

The monthly *Journal of the National Cancer Institute* presents original reports of cancer research by scientists around the world. Other NCI publications include the *Monograph Series* for proceedings of scientific meetings and other lengthy reports, and *Cancer Chemotherapy Reports*. *Carcinogenesis Abstracts* and *Cancer Therapy Abstracts* contain short summaries of articles appearing in thousands of scientific journals. A great variety of periodic and special reports, computerized data banks and conferences, workshops and seminars provide additional ways to speed the flow of cancer information by NCI.

Office on Smoking and Health
Technical Information Center (TIC), HEW
Parklawn Building, Room 1-16
5600 Fishers Lane
Rockville, MD 20857
(301) 443-1690

Handicapping Conditions Served: Smoking-related health problems.

The Organization: Established in 1978, the Office of Smoking and Health (formerly the National Clearinghouse for Smoking and Health) is the U.S. Public Health Service program most concerned about the health hazards of smoking. Its Technical Information Center (TIC) collects, organizes, and disseminates the world's literature on smoking and its effects on health. TIC's scientific and technical collection comprises over 30,000 hard copy reports on all aspects of smoking and health. In addition, a bibliographic data base has more than 12,000 records in machine readable form. It is expected that this file will be greatly expanded over the next three years. During 1980, TIC's numerical data base will become operational. Survey research information from several smoking and health sources will be available through this service.

Information Services: Computer searches of TIC's bibliographic data base are performed upon request; users are asked to submit completed Search Request Forms, available from TIC. Both technical and public education publications may be obtained from the Center, and include the *Bibliography on Smoking and Health,* the *Directory of On-Going Research in Smoking and Health,* and the *Smoking and Health Bulletin,* a current awareness periodical listing references on all aspects of smoking and health. Current research from the Directory will be available in machine readable form, beginning in early 1980. Reprints of articles included in the *Bulletin* are available on a limited basis. There is no charge for TIC services and publications.

Program Research Associates
45 Maplewood Mall
Philadelphia, PA 19144
(215) 849-7095

Handicapping Conditions Served: Primarily developmental disabilities.

The Organization: Program Research Associates (PRA, formerly the EMC Institute) is a nonprofit organization established by a group of professionals experienced in the field of developmental disabilities and other areas of social programming. PRA was founded to provide research, systems development, and consultation in program planning, design, implementation, evaluation, administration, and management to public and private agencies at the national, regional, state, and local levels. For many years PRA has received grants and contracts from Bureau of Developmental Disabilities, Department of Health, Education, and Welfare, to formulate state planning guidelines for developmental disabilities programs, to provide technical assistance to states in developing their plans, and to design evaluation procedures for state developmental disabilities programs.

Information Services: In addition to providing technical assistance through government grants and contracts in the areas mentioned above, PRA has prepared issue papers pertinent to current program functions and planning trends, including extensive analysis of P.L. 95-602 (the Rehabilitation, Comprehensive Services, and Developmental Disabilities Amendments of 1978). Among the topics covered by these papers are the following: 1) the transition to P.L. 95-602; 2) the analysis of changes in the Rehabilitation Act of 1973; 3) probable changes in the developmental disabilities program; 4) coordination and case management in the developmental disabilities program; and 5) the definition of developmental disabilities given in P.L. 95-602, including estimates of this population. Issue papers on prevalence rates for developmental disabilities as defined in P.L. 94-103 (Developmentally Disabled Assistance and Bill of Rights Act) and needs assessment and program data under the Act are also available. There is a charge for these publications.

Project PAVE
Parents' Campaign for Handicapped
 Children and Youth
Box 1492
Washington, DC 20013
(202) 833-4160

Handicapping Conditions Served: All handicapping conditions.

The Organization: Funded under a contract with the U.S. Office of Education's Bureau of Education for the Handicapped and the Office for Civil Rights, Department of Health, Education, and Welfare, Project PAVE (Parents Advocating for Vocational Education) is conducted by the Parents' Campaign for Handicapped Children and Youth, a nonprofit organization of parents which advocates for the rights of disabled children and works closely with local parent groups throughout the country. Initiated in 1978, Project PAVE conducts seminars in various locations across the country to train parents and disabled youth as advocates who can intervene on behalf of handicapped high school students in need of vocational education. Project PAVE's staff provides technical assistance to the trained advocates after the seminars and continues to work with sponsoring local groups to bring about compliance of local education agencies with relevant federal and state laws and to develop new vocational education options.

Information Services: Information on PAVE training sites and local advocate groups in these areas is available from the Project. Inquirers may also obtain information on pertinent legislation, referral to vocational education resource centers, and a bibliography. There is no charge for this information.

Project SHARE
National Clearinghouse for Improving
 the Management of Human Services
P.O. Box 2309
Rockville, MD 20852
(301) 428-0700

Handicapping Conditions Served: All handicaps.

The Organization: Established in 1975, Project Share (National Clearinghouse for Improving the Management of Human Services) compiles and disseminates information on human services planning, administration, and evaluation to human services managers. The Project is operated by the Aspen Systems Corporation for the Office of the Assistant Secretary for Planning and Evaluation, Department of Health, Education, and Welfare.

Information Services: Users may request searches of Project Share's bibliographic data base, which includes records of documents on services integration, model programs, cost analysis, records management, and compliance with federal regulations. Copies of most documents cited, which include working papers, project descriptions, manuals, feasibility studies, conference proceedings, and reports prepared by federal, state, and local government agencies, government contractors, and national associations, are available from the Project or the National Technical Information Service (see separate entry). Sources for other documents are clearly indicated in the printout which also gives descriptive abstracts of each publication. Among topics of interest to professionals in the handicapped field are the following: deinstitutionalization, normalization of the lives of chronically ill and disabled persons, alternate care, advocacy, and transportation services for handicapped persons.

The *Journal of Human Services Abstracts*, published quarterly by the Project, is an indexed list of document input into the data base. It is restricted to items acquired by the Clearinghouse and is not meant to provide comprehensive coverage of the field.

Project Share also publishes the following: 1) a series of monographs which survey the literature and state of the art in various areas of human services planning and management; 2) annotated bibliographies of Project Share materials on selected topics of major interest to human services planners and managers; 3) comprehensive summaries of major documents in the Project collection; and 4) a newsletter which highlights social services and information programs, new publications, and current research problems, and announces selected national meetings of interest to readers.

The Project's reference service provides individuals and organizations with information on any topic within the scope of the Project. In addition to customized bibliographies generated from the Project's data base, inquirers may receive manually prepared citations and referrals to other organizations.

There is no charge for the Project's Services. Government agencies, educational institutions, and libraries may obtain complimentary subscriptions to Project Share publications. Individuals and for profit organizations may subscribe to the *Journal of Human Services Abstracts* through the National Technical Information Service; they may request the newsletter, *Sharing*, directly from the Clearinghouse.

Psychological Abstracts Information
Services
American Psychological Association
1200 17th Street, N.W.
Washington, DC 20036
(800) 336-4980 (except Washington, DC, and Virginia)
(202) 833-5908 (Washington, DC, and Virginia)

Handicapping Conditions Served: All handicaps.

The Organization: Part of the American Psychological Association, a professional society of psychologists and educators, Psychological Abstracts Information Services (PsycINFO) is a family of interrelated information services providing a variety of ways to access the world's published literature in psychology and related behavioral and social sciences.

Information Services: PsycINFO publishes the *Psychological Abstracts (PA)* journal, a comprehensive monthly compilation of nonevaluative summaries of the world's scientific literature in psychology and related disciplines. Each year PsycINFO scans materials from over 1,000 periodicals and about 1,500 books, technical reports, and monographs for inclusion in *PA*. Among the 16 major classification categories according to which abstracts are grouped are the following: "Physical and Psychological disorders," "Psychometrics," "Treatment and Prevention," and "Educational Psychology," which includes special education. Documents on the characteristics of physically and psychologically disabled populations and their treatment may be found under these classification categories. *PA's Volume Index*, a subject and author index, is published twice yearly; cumulative indexes from 1969-71, 1972-74, and 1975-77 are available. Beginning in 1980, *PsycScan Clinical Psychology* and *PsycSCAN Developmental Psychology* will publish quarterly selected abstracts contained in the *PA* monthly journal.

Computer searches of *PA* from 1967, a file containing nearly 300,000 items, may be ordered from PsycINFO. Approximately 26% of the documents included in this on-line data base concern characteristics of physically and psychologically impaired persons and their treatment. In addition, about 13% of the documents in the data base are on educational research; items on handicapped students form a subset of these records. Many of the terms used by PsycINFO's information specialists to search this file are related to specific handicapping conditions and treatment, including physical and mental disorders; attitudes towards mental illness, mental retardation, physical handicaps, and sensory handicaps; rehabilitation; and special education and mainstreaming. These keywords are listed in the *Thesaurus of Psychological Index Terms* which may be purchased from PsycINFO.

Descriptions of PsycINFO services and price information are available upon request. Direct on-line access to the PsycINFO data base may be arranged through Bibliographic Retrieval Services, the System Development Corporation, or Lockheed (see Data Base Vendors, page 97).

Research to Prevent Blindness, Inc.
(RPB)
598 Madison Avenue
New York, NY 10022
(212) 752-4333

Handicapping Conditions Served: Blindness and visual impairments.

The Organization: Research to Prevent Blindness provides financial support to ophthalmology departments of 50 U.S. medical schools for the purpose of scientific research on the causes, prevention, diagnosis and treatment of diseases causing blindness. It has supported the development of techniques such as laser treatment, vitrectomy, microsurgery and therapeutic use of contact lenses as well as extensive basic studies of the eye and its diseases. Incentives are provided to attract outstanding scientists to eye research through annual awards.

Information Services: RPB provides information concerning vision research to news media, legislators, practicing ophthalmologists and the public. The RPB National Science Writers Seminar in Eye Research, conducted every several years, brings together outstanding vision scientists, news editors and writers for reports and discussions of progress in the management and prevention of blinding eye diseases. RPB publishes the formal scientific reports for dissemination to the nation's practicing eye physicians. RPB answers general inquiries about eye research on a limited basis. It does not offer specific advice or recommendations on individual eye problems. All applications for support of vision research must be made through chairmen of departments of ophthalmology.

Science and Education Administration
Technical Information Systems, USDA
National Agricultural Library Building
Beltsville, MD 20705
(301) 344-3704

Handicapping Conditions Served: All handicapping conditions.

The Organization: The Scientific and Education Administration (SEA) was established by the Secretary of Agriculture in 1978 to improve the nationwide effectiveness of research, teaching, and information dissemination in the food and agricultural sciences. SEA reflects the consolidation of the former Extension Service, the National Agricultural Library, and other UDSA agencies.

AGRICOLA (Agricultural OnLine Access), a family of data bases developed by SEA and its cooperators, indexes books, reports, and approximately 6,000 journals in agriculture-related fields, including food and nutrition. AGRICOLA contains more than one million citations, several hundred of which refer to documents on various aspects of handicapping conditions, for example, nutrition for disabled persons, independent living, and work experiences programs for handicapped individuals.

Information Services: Online access to AGRICOLA is available through Lockheed, the System Development Corporation, and Bibliographic Retrieval Services (see Data Base Vendors, page 97). Copies of most documents in AGRICOLA searches may be obtained from SEA's Technical Information Systems for a nominal photocopying fee. Libraries may borrow books which are not classified as reference materials or rare books.

**Sex Information and Education Council
of the U.S. (SIECUS)
84 Fifth Avenue
New York, NY 10011
(212) 929-2300**

Handicapping Conditions Served: All handicaps.

The Organization: SIECUS has as its stated purpose the promotion of free access to full and accurate information on all aspects of sexuality, as every person's basic right. Most of the organization's work is directed to the general population. However, some material is geared to special audiences: teens, their parents, the physically and mentally handicapped, and the aging. SIECUS is helping to stimulate hospital programs to assure the handicapped help with their problems of sexuality.

Information Services: SIECUS has several information and education functions: to act as a clearinghouse for information on materials and other organizations with information on sexuality; as a referral service for anyone needing help; as a consultant on planning of programs in institutional and community settings; as a publisher of original books, study guides, and specialized bibliographies, and the *SIECUS Report*; as a reference and research source; and as a sponsor of symposia nationally and worldwide.

In 1978, SIECUS became affiliated with New York University's Department of Health Education (School of Education, Health, Nursing, and Arts Professions). The SIECUS Library, a collection of 15 years of scientific literature on sexuality, is now housed at NYU.

SIECUS publications include:

• *A Resource Guide in Sex Education for the Mentally Retarded*, produced in conjunction with the American Association for Health, Physical Education, and Recreation;

• *Developing Community Acceptance of Sex Education for the Mentally Retarded;*

• *A Bibliography of Resources in Sex Education for the Mentally Retarded;*

• *Sex Education and Family Life for Visually Handicapped Children and Youth: A Resource Guide,* cosponsored by the American Federation for the Blind;

• *Selective Bibliography on Sex and the Handicapped;*

• *Human Sexuality: A Selected Bibliography for Professionals;*

• *Human Sexuality: Books for Everyone*; and

• *SIECUS Report*, a bimonthly newsletter (for professionals and laypersons) with articles, reviews of current works, and important news in the field. The May 1976 issue dealt entirely with "The Handicapped and Sexual Health." In March 1979, two articles appeared in the newsletter which dealt with sexuality and the handicapped.

In addition to publications, SIECUS will answer lay and professionals inquiries by phone or by letter (if self-addressed, stamped envelope is included with the request).

**Smithsonian Science Information
Exchange**
1730 M Street, N.W.
Washington, DC 20036
(202) 381-4211

Handicapping Conditions Served: All handicaps.

The Organization: Established in 1969 as the Medical Sciences Information Exchange, the Smithsonian Science Information Exchange (SSIE) collects, indexes, stores, and disseminates data about ongoing research projects in the social, life, and physical sciences. Information on basic and applied research in progress is collected for more than 1300 federal, state, and local agencies, foundations, universities, and other organizations. Most of the projects in the SSIE file are sponsored by the Federal Government. Since registration of documents is voluntary, most, but not all, federally funded research is included. SSIE's active file, which covers material collected during the past two government fiscal years, contains information on more than 200,000 current and recently completed research projects. New project information is added to the file daily; records for projects continuing over a period of years are updated annually. The current file contains records for more than 20,000 projects in all areas of the social and behavioral sciences.

Information Services: In response to individual requests, staff specialists search the SSIE data base for research projects on specific subjects. Searches for projects from particular performing organizations or departments, specific geographic areas, or for any combination of similar requirements can also be made. Project notices in the file can be identified by any subject or administrative index code assigned to them. The subject specialist who conducts the search reviews the results to assure relevancy of project notices, and, if necessary, contacts the user for clarification of his or her information needs. Output received by the user contains essential information about each project, including the supporting organization, the performing organization, the principal and coinvestigators, the time period covered by the project notices, and, in most cases, a 200 word description of the work to be performed. Information on handicapped persons falls principally in the following categories: employment, education, transportation, psychological and social adjustment, barrier-free design, rehabilitation engineering, and medical research. Estimates of the costs for individual custom searches are available without charge.

Prepared searches on subjects of high current interest are also available. Inquirers may request free brochures listing published searches in various subject areas, including social sciences, behavior sciences, and engineering, all of which list searches on various aspects of handicapping conditions and related services. In addition, both standard and custom selected dissemination of information is available, providing subscribers with regular updates of new additions to the SSIE data base on topics of interest to them.

The *SSIE Science Newsletter*, for which there is a subscription fee, contains articles of interest to the scientific community and information on new prepared searches.

The SSIE data base is available on-line through Bibliographic Retrieval Services, Lockheed, and the System Development Corporation (see Data Base Vendors, page 97).

Sociological Abstracts, Inc. (SA)
P.O. Box 22206
San Diego, CA 92122
(714) 565-6603

Handicapping Conditions Served: All handicaps.

The Organization: Founded in 1953 by a group of sociologists, Sociological Abstracts (SA) has continued to provide nonevaluative abstracts from relevant journal literature in sociology and related disciplines. Journal articles from 1963 to the present are produced in both paper copy and machine readable form. SA's collection contains material on the sociological aspects of handicapping conditions, including major diseases, mental illness, and physical disabilities.

Information Services: Researchers, administrators, and other users may obtain custom searches of SA, including searches of pre-1963 records, and of related data bases. Cost estimates for these searches may be prepared in advance without obligation.

In addition to *Sociological Abstracts*, SA's major subscription journal, *Language and Language Behavior Abstracts* is also available on a subscription basis. This journal is devoted to linguistics and related disciplines, and its contents may be searched by SA.

The following publications are also available from SA: *International Review of Publications in Sociology*, which lists sociology books and book reviews published in sociology journals; microfiches of unpublished papers; *Supplements*, containing abstracts of papers presented at regional, national, and international meetings of sociologists; and *Social Welfare, Social Policy, and Social Development*, SA's new publication of nonevaluative abstracts in the three title areas.

Searches of the *Sociological Abstracts* and *Language and Language Behavior Abstracts* files are available on-line through Lockheed (see Data Base Vendors, page 97).

Tel-Med, Inc.
National Headquarters
22700 Cooley Drive
Colton, CA 92324
(714) 825-6034

Handicapping Conditions Served: All handicaps.

The Organization: Tel-Med is a library of tape-recorded health care messages, which are disseminated nationwide to over 250 hospitals, medical societies, universities, and other agencies that are licensed to sponsor Tel-Med programs. Licensees set up telephone lines to communicate taped messages to the public. An individual calls, selects a tape, and an operator plays the appropriate message. The 3 to 5 minute tapes are written by physicians and other health care specialists, and are reviewed periodically to insure that the most current information on the subject is contained. Tapes are also reviewed by local community medical boards of the sponsoring agents.

Information Services: Tel-Med's library consists of more than 300 tapes on health care subjects. Of specific interest to the handicapped are Tel-Med's series of tapes on diabetes, eye care and hearing, and cancer. Tel-Med also produces tapes on arthritis-rheumatism, cleft lip and palate, cystic fibrosis, muscular dystrophy, sickle cell anemia, multiple sclerosis, brain damage recovery, social security, and SSI and state disability insurance. Selection of tapes available varies among licensees.

Tel-Med sends organizational brochures, including information on licensing procedures, and a list of Tel-Med licensees, upon request. Tel-Med publishes a newsletter for licensees and will provide them with copies of resources used to document the tapes.

Therapeutic Recreation Information Center (TRIC)
Department of Physical Education and Recreation
University of Colorado
Box 354
Boulder, CO 80309
(303) 492-7333

Handicapping Conditions Served: All handicaps.

The Organization: TRIC is a computer based information acquisition, storage, retrieval, and dissemination center specifically concerned with published and unpublished materials related to recreation services to ill, disadvantaged, disabled, and aging persons. The TRIC computerized data base of more than 2,000 indexed items, which was developed in 1971 at Columbia University, is updated as needed. TRIC also maintains a comprehensive on-site library of information materials, and provides consultation services to individuals and organizations for recreation inservice education and training projects.

Information Services: TRIC provides computer printouts containing annotated bibliographic reference materials (abstracts) on specific topics related to recreation for special populations. Abstract printouts are categorized in major and minor files, depending on the number of abstracts included in the descriptor files. Major topic files related to the handicapped include those titled "disabled," "mentally retarded," "physically disabled," "rehabilitation," "research-reports," "camping," and "children." TRIC information processing specialists select appropriate major or minor files for the user based on the specific problem description made by the inquirer. Fees for TRIC searches are based on the number of abstracts contained in the particular file or files requested.

TRIC's services are available to educators, researchers, students, practitioners, or others interested in therapeutic recreation for special groups or individuals in need of services. For additional information about TRIC, contact Dr. Fred Martin.

Data Base Vendors

Three major commercial organizations that offer access to on-line data bases are described below. These on-line data bases contain machine-readable records which give bibliographic information on documents in defined subject areas. A user's computer terminal is linked to the vendor's computer system via telephone allowing a user to search selected data bases in an interactive mode. A search strategy, formed by combining key words (or subject descriptors), is used to scan the data base. Documents of interest may be displayed for review, or printed off-line (saving expensive connect-time) and mailed.

The organizations listed offer training courses in using the data bases.

Bibliographic Retrieval Services, Inc. (BRS)
Corporation Park, Building 702
Scotia, NY 12302
(518) 374-5011
(800) 833-4707 (Outside New York)

Bibliographic Retrieval Services (BRS) provides access to approximately 30 data bases for on-line searching; for some of these, BRS is the only commercial vendor. Data bases of particular interest to professionals in the handicapped field are listed in the table at the end of this section. The larger data bases permit on-line searches of current documents (three to five years old) and off-line processing of earlier materials.

Charges for BRS searches include subscription fees, royalties for some data bases, telecommunication fees, and off-line print and search charges. The *BRS System Reference Manual*, containing information on all BRS data bases, and *Searching the Medlars Data Base* may be purchased from BRS.

Lockheed Information Systems
Department 50-20, Building 201
3251 Hanover Street
Palo Alto, CA 94304
(800) 982-5838 (California)
(800) 227-1960 (Outside California)

Lockheed's DIALOG retrieval service allows access to more than 100 data bases, some of which are available only through Lockheed. The DIALOG data bases containing information on various aspects of disabling conditions and services to handicapped individuals are listed in a table at the end of this section.

Prices for data base searches vary and are based on computer connect time, use of one or two data communications networks, and off-line printing of records. During the first month of service, users receive a credit of up to $100 for computer connect time. The Lockheed pricing schedule also offers discounts based upon the quantity of work to be performed and contractual arrangements.

The *Data Base Catalog*, which describes available files, and the *Subject Guide to DIALOG Databases* are available at no charge. The following may be purchased: *Guide to DIALOG Databases* (three volumes), *A Brief Guide to DIALOG Searching,* and *DIALIST Merged Indexes*. In addition, a list of aids (thesauri, subject classification lists, journal listings, search guides, etc.) supplied by data base originators is available.

SDC Search Service
System Development Corporation
2500 Colorado Avenue
Santa Monica, CA 90406
(800) 352-6689 (California)
(800) 421-7229 (Outside California)

Through ORBIT (On-Line Retrieval of Bibliographic Text), SDC's retrieval system, the user may access more than 50 data bases, many of which are available exclusively through SDC. The SDC files which reference documents on handicapping conditions and programs for disabled persons are listed in a table at the end of this section.

The fee structure for SDC's Search Service has three elements: computer time, usage of a telecommunications network, and off-line printing of citations. Discounts are applied automatically to accounts which use the system for at least five hours in any given month.

Copies of original documents from selected SDC data bases, including ERIC and NTIS, may be ordered on-line; document suppliers then forward copies of requested reports and articles to the user. Charges for documents vary according to the supplier and the length of the article.

Consultation with information professionals is available free of charge via the toll-free numbers listed above. SDC staff responds to systems questions and advises on search strategies and which data bases to use.

Literature describing the SDC Search Service, including descriptions of ORBIT's data bases, is available free of charge. A complimentary copy of the *Quick Reference Guide*, a desk-top reference tool giving concise information on the system and data bases, is supplied to users; additional copies may be purchased. The *Basic ORBIT User Manual* and microform indexes listing subject terms for each file may also be purchased.

Data Bases Available from Major Data Base Vendors

	BRS	Lockheed	SDC
AGRICOLA (see Science and Education Administration)	X	X	X
Comprehensive Dissertation Index (see Dissertation Information Services)	X	X	X
Conference Papers Index		X	X
Educational Resources Information Clearinghouse (ERIC)	X	X	X
Exceptional Child Education (see Council for Exceptional Children)	X	X	
Excerpta Medica		X	
Medlars (see National Library of Medicine)	X		
National Information Center for Special Education Materials (NISCEM)	X	X	
National Institute of Mental Health (NIMH) (see National Clearinghouse for Mental Health Information)	X		
National Rehabilitation Information Center (NARIC) (available mid-1980)	X		
National Technical Information Service (NTIS)	X	X	X
Psychological Abstracts	X	X	X
Smithsonian Science Information Exchange (SSIE)	X	X	X
Social Science Citation Index (see Institute for Scientific Information)	X	X	X
Sociological Abstracts		X	
TRIS-On-Line (see Highway Research Information Service). TRIS-On-Line includes the HRIS data base and additional material on transportation		X	

Part Three

FEDERAL GOVERNMENT OTHER THAN INFORMATION UNITS

**Committee for Purchase from the Blind
and Other Severely Handicapped**
2009 14th Street North, Suite 610
Arlington, VA 22201
(703) 557-1145

Handicapping Conditions Served: Blindness and severe handicaps.

The Organization: This presidentially-appointed Committee was established to set up the rules and regulations necessary to carry out the provisions of the Javits-Wagner-O'Day Act. The Committee directs the procurement of selected commodities and services by the Federal Government to qualified workshops serving the blind and other severely handicapped individuals with the objective of increasing employment opportunities of these individuals. **National Industries for the Blind** and **National Industries for the Severely Handicapped** (see separate entries), which represent qualified workshops, submit requests for new products and services, and the Committee determines their suitability.

Information Services: All inquiries are referred to the appropriate workshop representative: National Industries for the Blind or National Industries for the Severely Handicapped (see separate entries).

**Community Services Administration
  (CSA)**
1200 19th Street N.W.
Washington, DC 20506
(202) 254-5840

Handicapping Conditions Served: All handicaps.

The Organization: The Community Services Administration is an independent Federal agency which funds local community action agencies through its regional offices. More than 870 community action agencies provide a variety of services (depending on the agency), including vocational and psychological counseling, to persons whose incomes fall below the Federal poverty level. Indigent handicapped persons are included in the populations that the agencies serve. CSA's pilot and demonstration projects in the handicapped area have been devoted to the accessibility of local agencies.

Information Services: CSA provides technical assistance booklets to grantees and other interested persons on making facilities accessible at low cost. A directory of technical assistance consultants, listed by state, is also available. For information about local services or referrals to health care providers, contact local community action agencies.

**Administration for Public Services
  (APS)
Office of Human Development Services,
  HEW**
Room 2006, Switzer Building
330 C Street, S.W.
Washington, DC 20201
(202) 245-0222

Handicapping Conditions Served: All handicaps.

The Organization: The Administration for Public Services (APS) administers the Federal/state social services program authorized by Title XX of the Social Security Act. State programs vary, being shaped primarily by the need and priorities of the individual states. APS provides oversight, leadership, and technical assistance on planning, coordination, and delivery of services. Within a state's annual authorization, APS funds 90 percent of a state's family planning expenditures and 75 percent of other Title XX program expenditures. The law requires that at least half of the Federal payment be spent on services to welfare recipients, and that each state provide at least three services to the indigent blind, aged or disabled. Representative state services include information and referral, day care, counseling, transportation, homemaker, health-related, vocational rehabilitation, protective, and foster care services. State social service programs are operated in the 50 states, the District of Columbia, Guam, Puerto Rico, and the Virgin Islands.

Information Services: General program information pamphlets and statistical reports are available through the HDS Office of Public Affairs, Room 329D, 200 Independence Ave., S.W., Washington, DC 20201 (202) 472-7257.

Architectural and Transportation Barriers
   Compliance Board (A&TBCB)
330 C Street, S.W., Room 1010
Washington, DC 20201
(202) 245-1591 (Voice/TTY)

This office will be transferred to the Department of Education. Address changes will be announced in Programs for the Handicapped. *You may wish to request notification by sending the self-mailer card inserted in the Directory.*

Handicapping Conditions Served: All handicaps.

The Organization: The Architectural and Transportation Barriers Compliance Board (A&TBCB) was created by Section 502 of the Rehabilitation Act of 1973 to enforce the Architectural Barriers Act of 1968 (P.L. 90-480) which requires that most buildings and facilities designed, constructed, altered, or leased by the Federal Government since 1969 be accessible to handicapped persons. As the Federal agency established to monitor P.L. 90-480, the Board is responsible for ensuring that all waivers and modifications are consistent with the Act, and for developing minimum guidelines and requirements for standards issued by other Federal agencies under the Act. The Board handles complaints about inaccessible facilities through its Executive Director. Only written complaints are accepted. The complainant's name is not disclosed without written consent. The Board may conduct investigations, hold public hearings, and issue orders to comply with the Act. Among the Board's responsibilities is the planning for accessible transportation and housing for handicapped persons; this involves cooperation with other agencies, organizations, and individuals also working toward such goals. The Board is also responsible for exploring communication barriers, and for making administrative and legislative recommendations.

Information Services: Publications to educate the general public on the mission of the Board are available free of charge. Sample titles are: *About Barriers* and *Access America: The Architectural Barriers Act and You*. The Board answers technical information questions from complainants and builders, and handles general information questions on ramps and other methods of designing accessible homes and commercial facilities.

Bureau of Developmental Disabilities (BDD)
Office of Human Development Services, HEW
Room 3070, Switzer Building
Washington, DC 20201
(202) 245-0335

Handicapping Conditions Served: Developmental disabilities including mental retardation. The handicap must originate before age 22, be expected to continue indefinitely, and constitute a major handicap in several areas of life's functioning.

The Organization: The Bureau of Developmental Disabilities Office (BDD) is responsible for administering the provisions of the Developmental Disabilities Assistance and Bill of Rights Act (P.L. 95-102) which became law in 1978. The Act makes available a range of strategies to meet the problems of developmentally disabled persons in terms of strengthening services and safeguarding individual rights. The Developmental Disabilities Office administers: formula grants to states for planning and administering programs, and delivering services to developmentally disabled persons; special project grants to improve the quality of services and programs, and for technical assistance and training of specialized personnel; and grants to university affiliated facilities which operate demonstration facilities for services to the developmentally disabled and for interdisciplinary training of specialized personnel. In addition, the Act authorized the establishment of Protection and Advocacy units for developmentally disabled people in each state, to assure that they obtain their rights and quality services.

Information Services: Information available from BDD relates to the programs it administers and is geared to officials of training and service agencies and facilities. Specific information regarding state services may be obtained from individual state agencies which operate developmental disabilities programs; for the names of state agencies, contact BDD.

**Bureau of Education for the
   Handicapped (BEH)
Office of Education, HEW
400 Maryland Ave., S.W.
Washington, DC 20202
(202) 245-2709**

This office will be transferred to the Department of Education, Office of Special Education and Rehabilitative Services within the next few months. Address changes will be announced in Programs for the Handicapped. *You may wish to request notification by sending the self-mailer card inserted in the Directory.*

Handicapping Conditions Served: All handicaps.

The Organization: The Bureau of Education for the Handicapped (BEH) is the principal agency for developing Federal policy, programs, and projects relating to the education and training of handicapped individuals. It deals primarily with state agencies of education and with institutions of higher learning which receive BEH grants for research and development of model programs in special education. BEH supplies funds and technical assistance to develop new and better methods and materials, and to disseminate these to all State Education Agencies (SEAs). Local education districts are the prime contact points for families of handicapped children. BEH has four divisions:

The **Division of Innovation and Development (DID)** supports research, demonstration, and evaluation activities in priority areas relating to education of handicapped children. The Division's largest demonstration activity is in early childhood with projects in every state to develop excellent service models. On request, local school districts can get permission from DID to replicate successful projects. Model programs are disseminated through the National Diffusion Network.

The **Division of Personnel Preparation (DPP)** administers a grant program and provides technical assistance to colleges and universities that train special education teachers, administrators, and parents and volunteers who have a special interest in educating handicapped children. The Division is responsible for inservice and preservice activities for regular and special educators, and new school personnel who interact with students in the least restrictive environment appropriate for them.

The **Division of Assistance to States (DAS)** works with state and local education offices to plan and improve programs for educating all handicapped children. Funds for BEH are allocated among the states to assist their special education programs and to implement P.L. 94-142, the Education for All Handicapped Children Act.

The **Division of Media Services (DMS)** develops and disseminates educational technology through its two branches. The *Learning Resources Branch* provides assessment and educational programming for children ages 0-21 through 15 Regional Resource Centers. The centers offer extensive materials, inservice training, and special education workshops for teachers interested in learning what is essential for good evaluation and placement of a handicapped child. The *Captioned Films and Telecommunications Branch* provides media and technology for the deaf through 60 depositories of educational films for the deaf in SEAs. Films are loaned free to schools and teaching personnel. A major activity sponsored by this branch is the National Captioning Institute (see separate entry), which provides captioned T.V. activities for deaf and hearing impaired audiences.

Information Services: Information activities on specific projects are disseminated by the individual projects which BEH supports throughout the country. Inquiries about local education services for the handicapped are referred to Closer Look, a BEH funded project (see separate entry). BEH handles inquiries from state agencies and educators about its own activities and funding; it does this through the four divisions: DID provides information regarding funds for research and development projects involving children ages 0-21; DPP provides information regarding personnel preparation funding and higher education training programs; DAS responds to complaints from parents and from educators on policy and problems with the system; and the DMS provides technical materials to local and state agencies for use in public and special schools. Dissemination of materials is also done through other BEH funded projects, such as the National Information Center for Special Education Materials (NICSEM) in Southern California (see separate entry) and the National Captioning Institute (see separate entry).

Additional information on specific dissemination activities conducted by individual projects can be obtained through the projects' officers. For general information about the division's activities, contact each division, telephone (202) 245-2727.

Crippled Children's Services
Office of Maternal and Child Health
Bureau of Community Health Services, HEW
5600 Fishers Lane, Room 7-39
Rockville, MD 20857
(301) 443-2170

Handicapping Conditions Served: All handicaps.

The Organization: Crippled Children's Services provides formula grants to states for direct medical and related services to crippled children. Other funding activities include: project grants to institutions of higher learning for training doctors, nurses, social workers, therapists, etc.; research grants for applied research programs in the field of maternal and child health; and special project grants for innovative demonstration projects of regional or national significance.

Information Services: The office provides information about its funding programs to lay and professional inquiries. A booklet, *Services to Crippled Children*, is available upon request. Since each state has its own plan for service tailored to their constituents' needs, information about direct services can best be obtained from each state's Crippled Children's Services.

Health Care Financing Administration
   (HCFA)
U.S. Department of Health, Education,
   and Welfare
Room 5221 Switzer Building
330 C Street, S.W.
Washington, DC 20201
(202) 245-0381

Handicapping Conditions Served: All handicaps.

The Organization: The Health Care Financing Administration (HCFA) was created in 1977 to oversee two major Federal medical assistance programs, Medicare and Medicaid, and related Federal medical quality control programs. HCFA administers funds for the Medicare program and the Federal portion of the Medicaid program. Medicare provides health insurance to persons over 65 and to disabled persons under 65 who meet the disability insurance (SSDI) requirements (see separate entry for the Social Security Administration) or who have permanent kidney failure.

Medicaid is a joint Federal/state program which provides health care services to persons with low incomes. Disabled persons may be eligible for Medicaid on the basis of their incomes. Because eligibility is determined by each state's program of public assistance (welfare) on the basis of broad Federal guidelines, there are geographic differences between eligibility requirements and types of service covered. Medicaid services are available in all states (except Arizona) and in Guam, Puerto Rico, and the Virgin Islands.

Information Services: Although HCFA responds to public inquiries, most of its informational resources are directed to state or local program managers of Medicare and Medicaid services. HCFA recommends that inquiries about Medicare benefits be directed to local Social Security offices, and inquiries about Medicaid benefits be directed to state public assistance or Medicaid offices, which respectively determine eligibility for the programs.

HCFA publishes general information brochures about Medicare and Medicaid which are available from most local access points, but may be obtained from the national office. Titles include: *A Guide to Medicare, Medicaid and You*, and *Medicaid Makes the Difference*. Information about Federal regulations under Title XVIII (Medicare) and Title XIX (Medicaid) of the Social Security Act may be obtained from HCFA. Statistics related to Medicaid programs in each state are regularly updated and published in *Data on the Medicaid Program*. A chart of *Medicaid Services by State* displays a breakdown of services provided and categories of recipients in each participating locale.

National Institute of Handicapped Research
   (NIHR)
Office of Human Development Services, HEW
Room 3058, Switzer Building
330 C Street, S.W.
Washington, DC 20201
(202) 245-0565

This office will be transferred to the Department of Education, Office of Special Education and Rehabilitative Services within the next few months. Address changes will be announced in Programs for the Handicapped. *You may wish to request notification by sending the self-mailer card inserted in the Directory.*

Handicapping Conditions Served: All handicaps.

The Organization: The National Institute of Handicapped Research (NIHR) was established in November 1978 by Public Law 95-602. Its mandate is to provide a comprehensive and coordinated Federal approach to all government research programs germane to the needs of the handicapped population. With an overview of Federal research activities, NIHR is expected to influence research to be more responsive and more directed to the medical, social, educational, emotional, and other needs of the disabled. In addition, NIHR will evaluate the effectiveness and efficiency of existing service delivery systems and will conduct a demonstration and training program in international rehabilitation research.

At this writing, the Institute is preparing to become fully operational.

Information Services: NIHR will function as a clearinghouse of information on research and progress.

Office for Civil Rights
Office of the Secretary, HEW
330 Independence Ave., S.W.
Washington, DC 20201
(202) 245-6700

Portions of units in the Office for Civil Rights which handle discrimination against handicapped individuals and technical assistance to educational program recipients covered by 504 regulations will be transferred to the Department of Education within the next few months.

Handicapping Conditions Served: All handicaps.

The Organization: The Office for Civil Rights is responsible for investigating discrimination on the basis of race, color, age, national origin, religion, mental and physical handicaps, and sex in Federally assisted programs. Recipients of Federal funds include elementary and secondary schools, colleges and universities, health and social rehabilitation facilities, and state agencies. OCR has the responsibility, as mandated by Congress, to implement and enforce Section 504 of the Rehabilitation Act of 1973, which concerns discrimination on the basis of handicap. Section 504 is the first piece of civil rights legislation on equal access for the handicapped in the areas of programs, services, and employment. OCR has three offices which work on 504 related issues:

The **Handicapped Discrimination Branch** of the Office of Standards, Policy and Research writes policy and interprets existing legislation for HEW as it relates to Section 504. Its principal advisory role of interpretation is to HEW regional offices and to other government agencies.

The **Office of Program Review and Assistance** provides technical assistance to government agencies, recipients of Federal funds, and private disability organizations to promote voluntary compliance with 504 in the most cost-effective way. Technical assistance units are located in each of the ten HEW regional offices.

The **Office of Compliance and Enforcement** conducts periodic compliance reviews to insure that regulations, standards and guidelines are implemented in a uniform, effective and timely manner. Public complaints against funds recipients are investigated by the regional office.

Information Services: The **Office of Public Affairs** is the main source of printed material on 504. It answers inquiries from the public and funds recipients and refers inquiries to appropriate central or regional OCR offices. Fact sheets on definitions, regulations, policy statements and guidelines relating to Section 504 may be obtained from the office; some are available in recorded form. Pamphlets relating to 504 include: *Your Responsibilities as a Health and Social Service Provider, Your Responsibilities as a School or College Administrator,* and *Your Rights as a Disabled Person. A Training and Resource Directory for Teachers Servicing Handicapped Students (K-12)* contains state listings of agencies which provide inservice training, technical assistance and informational materials to teachers of the handicapped.

Office of Handicapped Concerns (OHC)
Office of Education, HEW
400 Maryland Ave., S.W., Room 4129
Washington, DC 20202
(202) 245-0873

This office will be transferred to the Department of Education. Address changes will be announced in Programs for the Handicapped. *You may wish to request notification by sending the self-mailer card inserted in this Directory.*

Handicapping Conditions Served: All handicaps.

The Organization: The Office of Handicapped Concerns (OHC) provides policy advice to change the programs and processes of the U.S. Office of Education to meet the needs of handicapped Americans. OHC develops links between the Office of Education (OE) and state education agencies, colleges, universities, organizations, and associations. The office mission is to improve educational services for disabled individuals through: a) identification of educational programs of interest to handicapped Americans; b) dissemination of information on OE policies which relate to handicapped citizens; and c) national, regional, and local meetings with organizations and individuals interested in the education of handicapped citizens. The Office serves as liaison to education managers with handicapped citizens and organizations. In the future the office will address the issue of removing barriers to the employment of handicapped persons in the educational system.

Information Services: All OHC services are free of charge. Presently the office provides information on OE programs, and refers disabled individuals who seek employment in OE to selected employment coordinators. Organizations concerned with the development of educational and employment policies of handicapped educators are encouraged to call the office for advisory or consultative services.

President's Committee on Mental
    Retardation (PCMR)
Washington, DC 20201
(202) 245-7634

Handicapping Conditions Served: Mental retardation.

The Organization: The President's Committee on Mental Retardation (PCMR) is a Federal agency that acts as advocate for the mentally retarded. Its interest are prevention, better services, the most unrestricted settings, public acceptance of the retarded, and full citizenship rights for this handicapped group.

Through preparation of major resource documents and through national publicity, PCMR keeps the needs of the mentally retarded before agencies and people that can help them: the President, the public, Federal and state agencies, and consumers and providers of services in the public and private sector.

PCMR reports regularly to the President, Cabinet Members, agency officials, and legislators on the nation's progress in dealing with mentally retarded persons.

Information Services: Inquiries to PCMR go to the Public Information Office. This Office provides publications free of charge, on a single copy basis. Sample titles are: *Mental Retardation and the Law; The Naive Offender;* and *International Directory of Mental Retardation Resources.* Lists of national organizations dealing with research and educational activities for the mentally retarded are also available.

Project Head Start
Administration for Children, Youth
    and Families
Office of Human Development
    Services, HEW
P.O. Box 1182
Washington, DC 20013
(202) 755-7700

Handicapping Conditions Served: All handicaps.

The Organization: Project Head Start is administered by the Administration for Children, Youth and Families, and authorized by the Economic Opportunity Amendments of 1978 (P.L. 95-568). The law requires that no less than 10 percent of enrollment opportunities in Head Start programs in each state be available for handicapped children and that services be provided to meet their special needs. HEW regional offices award grants to local public and private agencies for the purpose of operating Head Start programs in their communities. The programs serve 3-5 year olds in more than 1350 rural and urban areas throughout the U.S. and Trust Territories.

Information Services: Local Head Start programs are the main source of information about specific services and eligibility. General information about Head Start is available from the national office, and includes an annual report and a directory of local Head Start programs listed by state. Head Start produces a number of materials designed for professional workers in child care programs. These materials include program manuals on mainstreaming handicapped preschoolers who have visual, hearing, speech and language, mental retardation, health, orthopedic, learning, and emotional disorders. Materials for the child care professional can be obtained only from the Government Printing Office.

Rehabilitation Services Administration
    (RSA)
Office of Human Development Services, HEW
Switzer Building
Washington, DC 20201
(202) 245-0322

This office will be transferred to the Department of Education, Office of Special Education and Rehabilitative Services within the next few months. Address changes will be announced in Programs *for the* Handicapped. *You may wish to request notification by sending the self-mailer card inserted in the* Directory.

Handicapping Conditions Served: All handicaps.

The Organization: The Rehabilitation Services Administration (RSA) runs the federal-state vocational rehabilitation program, which provides services to disabled people to help them become employable. Five services are provided to the handicapped person who is potentially employable: a) evaluation, b) counseling, c) vocational training, d) medical services, and e) job placement.

RSA provides administrative support to state programs through the **Office of Program Operations** and the **Office of Program Development**. In the **Office of Program Operations**, the *Bureau for the Blind and Visually Handicapped* administers the Randolph-Sheppard Act under which blind persons operate vending facilities, programs for blind persons located in state vocational rehabilitation agencies, and the Helen Keller National Center for Deaf-Blind Youths and Adults in Sands Point, New York (see separate entry); and the *Bureau of Vocational Rehabilitation* is responsible for administering state vocational rehabilitation programs, providing guidance and technical assistance to the states on services to eligible handicapped clients.

The **Office of Program Development** administers RSA's training programs, projects for special populations (e.g., older blind persons, migrants, etc.) and demonstration programs such as Independent Living, Client Assistance, and Projects with Industry.

A third office in RSA, the **Office of Advocacy and Coordination**, works with disability interest groups to advocate service and general social improvements for disabled persons. It also serves to coordinate RSA's programs with those of other Federal, state, local, and private agencies.

Information Services: Personal inquiries to RSA are handled by the correspondence control unit (telephone: (202) 245-0261), where potential clients are referred to the state agency in the geographic area where the clients reside. The Office of Program Operations and its Bureaus provide information for administrators on their respective grants/projects areas. The Bureau for the Blind and Visually Handicapped has an outreach program which includes eight regional representatives under the supervision of the New York based Helen Keller National Center for Deaf-Blind Youths and Adults, where deaf-blind individuals receive rehabilitation evaluation, training, or job placement. The Bureau of Vocational Rehabilitation Operations answers questions of state vocational agencies on the eligibility process and administration of state programs including the establishment and improvement of rehabilitation facilities and the review of annual state plans.

Social Security Administration (SSA)
6401 Security Boulevard
Baltimore, MD 21235
(301) 594-7700

Handicapping Conditions Served: All handicaps.

The Organization: The Social Security Administration administers a national program of contributory social insurance which pays benefits when earnings stop or are reduced because a worker retires, dies, or becomes disabled. Disability insurance (SSDI) provides a partial replacement of monthly earnings to disabled persons who meet work requirements for eligibility. After 24 months of receiving benefits under SSDI, persons automatically qualify for hospital and medical insurance under Medicare. (Persons of any age who need kidney dialysis or kidney transplant for permanent kidney failure also may be eligible for Medicare. Medicare protection for these people starts with the third month after they begin maintenance dialysis. Under certain conditions, protection can begin earlier.)

Supplemental Security Income (SSI), a noncontributory program financed out of general Federal funds, is also administered by SSA. SSI provides monthly payments to indigent aged, blind, and disabled persons, without regard to prior employment.

More than 1300 local Social Security offices are responsible for processing applications and claims for SSDI and SSI programs; they also determine eligibility for Medicare, although Medicare claims are processed by independent contractors or carriers.

Information Services: Local Social Security offices are often the best access points for information about programs and eligibility. Some local offices operate Teleservice Centers (TSC) so that program information and applications can be obtained by phone. TSC service representatives refer callers to local offices when more detailed information is required. SSA publishes more than 100 booklets on its programs, including specialized programs for the disabled. These booklets and a *Medicare Handbook* are available from the local offices.

The **Office of Public Inquiries** (phone number above) responds to questions about SSDI and SSI programs, proposed legislation, actuarial and statistical figures and general information.

The **Office of Research and Statistics** conducts research on the following programs: old age, survivors, disability, SSI, aid to families with dependent children, and child support enforcement. Findings are published in a variety of technical publications including:

1) *Some Statistical Research Resources Available at the Social Security Administration.* Briefly describes the type of data available from SSA statistical records.

2) *Survey of Disabled and Non-Disabled Adults: 1972.* Series of reports based on data collected in personal interviews with disabled, non-disabled, and previously disabled adults. The study focuses on the extent to which disability affects the labor force activity of working-age adults, and examines the effects of disability on the distribution of income. Among the titles in the series are the following: *Functional Capacity Limitation and Disability, Employment and Work Adjustment of the Disabled, Effect of Disability on Unit Income,* and *Some Characteristics of Social Security Disability Beneficiaries and Severely Disabled Nonbeneficiaries.* (A 1974 follow-up survey is being prepared by SSA.)

3) *Work Disability in the United States: A Chartbook.* Charts depicting the prevalence of disability, demographic characteristics of the disabled, and their health and economic status, summarizing the highlights of the findings from the 1972 survey, described above.

For information about research and statistics publications, contact the office at 1875 Connecticut Avenue, N.W., Washington, DC 20009, (202) 673-5576.

Employment Standards Administration
and Employment and Training Administration
Department of Labor (DOL)
200 Constitution Ave., N.W.
Washington, DC 20210
(202) 523-6666

Handicapping Conditions Served: All handicaps.

The Organization: The Department of Labor (DOL) develops policy and implements legislation for all workers in the nation. It is responsible for the enforcement of laws that protect the safety, health, job, and pension rights of workers. Each of DOL's 10 regional offices deals with issues affecting American handicapped workers, and within the Department's units specialized services are being implemented for disabled individuals.

The **Employment Standards Administration (ESA)** of DOL administers programs such as the *Office of Federal Contract Compliance Programs*, which processes complaints of handicapped individuals in cases of employment discrimination by Federal contractors. Complaints can be filed personally or by an authorized representative of the complainant, at any of the 10 DOL Regional Offices. DOL intervenes only when the cases cannot be handled locally. The *Wage and Hour Division* authorizes subminimum wages under the Fair Labor Standards Act to prevent curtailment of opportunities for employment for handicapped individuals who would not be able to command the minimum wage. The *Division of Special Minimum Wages* administers the regulations governing the employment of handicapped clients in sheltered workshops, handicapped workers in industry, and employment of patient workers based on their individual productivity.

The *Office of Workers' Compensation Programs* administers three basic Federal workers' compensation laws, whereby Federal employees (if injured on the job) can apply for a continued salary and assistance with medical expenses. The Office also administers the Black Lung Act of 1972 for coal mine workers.

The **Employment and Training Administration (ETA)** of DOL includes the *U.S. Employment Service (USES)* and the *Comprehensive Employment Training Act Programs (CETA)*. *USES* has had a program serving handicapped people for many years. Agency goals for handicapped workers are equal opportunity for employment and equal pay in competition with other applicants; employment at the highest skills permitted by their occupational qualifications; satisfactory adjustment to their chosen occupations and work situations; and employment that will not endanger others or aggravate their own disabilities. *CETA* money goes to state and local governments to train and employ economically disadvantaged, unemployed, and underemployed persons, many of whom are handicapped. CETA services include jobs and/or on-the-job training or classroom training. CETA may also provide handicapped individuals with support services such as transportation, health care, and removal of employment barriers/discriminatory hiring practices by eliminating unrealistic qualifications requirements, or restructuring of jobs to accommodate handicaps. DOL regional offices provide administrative services in the above program areas.

Information Services: Inquiries about programs of the Employment Standards Administration should be addressed to: Director, ESA Office of Information and Consumer Affairs, NDOL, Room C 4331, 200 Constitution Ave., N.W., Washington, DC 20210. For more information on the CETA programs, contact the Employment Training Administration, Office of Information, 601 D Street, N.W., Washington, DC 20213. For information on specific local CETA programs, locate the prime sponsor in your area (it may be the mayor's, governor's, or county commissioner's office). If you cannot locate it, call the U.S. Employment Service in your state for prime sponsor locations.

The U.S. Employment Service has developed a series of interviewing guides (e.g., cerebral palsy, mental retardation) which can be obtained from: Department of Labor, Employment Training Administration, 601 D Street, N.W., Room 10225, Washington, DC 20213. Inquiries about jobs on the local level should be addressed to the local U.S. Employment Service.

President's Committee on Employment of the Handicapped (PCEH)
1111 20th Street, N.W., 6th Floor
Washington, DC 20210
(202) 653-5044

Handicapping Conditions Served: All handicaps.

The Organization: The President's Committee on Employment of the Handicapped (PCEH) serves an advocacy and public awareness role in fostering job opportunities for handicapped people. As part of this effort, PCEH works with autonomous committees on employment of the handicapped at state and local levels, as well as producing its own publications and services. The Committee has a leading role in establishing an acceptable climate in industry and labor towards hiring handicapped individuals.

PCEH has organized around the national committee, a number of subcommittees which deal with special topics, and cooperating governors' and mayors' committees. Also, PCEH has been a strong advocate in the areas of architectural accessibility and in education and social activities for handicapped youth. The Committee has produced sensitizing campaigns to educate the general public on the employment and physical mobility needs of the handicapped population.

Information Services: PCEH provides information primarily in the area of employment, and has published pamphlets on architectural accessibility and education for handicapped youth. General information is provided on the Committee's activities and selected materials published by PCEH are sent on request. All services are free.

Publications developed by PCEH are representative of the Committee's advocacy efforts. Some sample titles are: *Affirmative Action for Disabled People: A Pocket Guide*, a brief explanation of sections 503 and 504 of the Rehabilitation Act of 1973; *Dear Employer* and *Look Who's Minding the Store*, notes on current information on employing handicapped people; *Architectural Barriers Checklist*, a pamphlet which includes a guide for determining the accessibility of college and university facilities; *Bibliography of Secondary Materials for Teaching Handicapped Students*; and several guides on job placement for persons with specific disabilities. If a person needs information on how to get specific materials, the Committee's staff will help in locating the materials.

**Office of Independent Living for the
    Disabled (OILD)**
**Department of Housing and Urban
    Development**
451 7th Street, S.W., Room 9106
Washington, DC 20410
(202) 755-7366

Handicapping Conditions Served: All handicaps.

The Organization: The Office of Independent Living for the Disabled (OILD), established by the Department of Housing and Urban Development (HUD) in June 1977, is the focal point within the Departmental Headquarters for ensuring that the disabled are appropriately represented and addressed throughout all of HUD's programs and activities.

OILD develops and evaluates Departmental policies, standards, procedures, and guidelines for HUD programs in order to respond to the housing, community development, and related needs of people of all ages with physical, developmental, or mental disabilities. OILD initiates training and information programs that enable Federal, state, and local officials, housing and service providers, and disabled consumers to become more aware of the varying needs of the disabled and to identify the HUD programs that will allow full participation of disabled individuals in housing and community development.

Current projects of OILD include a Demonstration Program for the Deinstitutionalization of the Chronically Mentally Ill, a Congregate Housing Services Program, and HANDI-TAP (technical assistance program for the development of community housing for handicapped individuals). Also, OILD assists in the revision of the ANSI architectural accessibility standards and the development of HUD's Section 504 regulations dealing with non-discrimination on the basis of handicap in Federally assisted programs and activities.

Information Services: OILD staff responds to inquiries on projects funded by HUD that can benefit the disabled; for example, the Community Development Block Grant Program, Section 8 Rental Assistance Program, Section 235 Home Ownership Program, Independent Group Residences and Congregate Housing, Section 202 Direct Loans for Housing for the Elderly or Handicapped, Section 106(b) Seed Money, Public Housing, Management Contracts, Section 231 Mortgage Insurance (Housing for the Elderly or Handicapped), Mobile Loan Insurance Program, and other programs administered by HUD. OILD is not a granting or funding unit.

National Park Service
Department of the Interior
18th and C Street, N.W.
Washington, DC 20240
(202) 343-2161

Handicapping Conditions Served: All handicaps.

The Organization: The National Park Service administers the nation's national park system, including parks and natural, historical, recreational, and cultural areas and facilities.

Information Services: The Park Service accepts inquiries on all of its national park activities and facilities. Information is provided on camping and recreational facilities accessible to handicapped individuals. All information is free. The Office of Special Programs and Populations handles lay and professional inquiries on national park facilities for the handicapped. Also, the office offers technical assistance to service providers, and deals with policies and procedures for all special groups.

114

**Urban Mass Transportation Administration
    (UMTA)
Department of Transportation
400 Seventh Street, S.W.
Washington, DC 20590
(202) 426-4023**

Handicapping Conditions Served: All handicapped and elderly persons who are nonambulatory or semi-ambulatory and are unable, without special facilities or special planning or design, to utilize mass transportation facilities and services effectively.

The Organization: The Urban Mass Transportation Administration was established to assist in the development of improved mass transportation facilities, equipment, techniques, and methods; to encourage the planning and establishment of urban mass transportation systems; and to provide assistance to state and local governments in financing such systems. In addition, UMTA is responsible for the enforcement of Section 504 regulations as they apply to mass transportation grantees. UMTA provides limited funding for research studies to identify handicapped populations, their transportation needs, and accessibility of existing mass transportation systems. Several types of grants are available to transportation agencies to improve services to the handicapped and elderly. For example, one UMTA program provides funds to nonprofit organizations to purchase vans to transport the handicapped and elderly.

Information Services: Most information provided by UMTA is directed to transit operators. The ten regional offices of UMTA are the best sources of information for local providers. The Public Affairs office headquarters (telephone number above) will direct inquiries to the appropriate national or regional office. Information about UMTA's program of assistance to nonprofit organizations is available from state departments of transportation. Handicapped persons who need information about local services are advised to contact local transportation authorities.

UMTA sponsored studies and surveys are published by the National Technical Information Service (NTIS) and are available from NTIS or the Transportation Research Board (TRB) of the National Academy of Sciences (see separate entries for NTIS and TRB). Publications available from UMTA include *Elderly and Handicapped Transportation: Local Government Approaches*, and *Transportation Assistance for Elderly and Handicapped Persons*.

**National Audiovisual Center
National Archives and Records Service
General Services Administration
Washington, DC 20409
(301) 763-1896**

Handicapping Conditions Served: All handicapping conditions.

The Organization: The National Audiovisual Center was created in 1969 to serve the public by making federally produced audiovisual materials available for use through distribution services and by serving as the central clearinghouse for all U.S. Government audiovisual materials. Through the Center's distribution programs, the public has access to audiovisual materials covering a variety of subjects, which include rehabilitation, special education, and health and medicine, including treatment of stroke, cancer, spinal cord injuries, arthritis, alcoholism, drug abuse, and other disabling conditions.

Many of the Center's audiovisual materials are for general use, while others are designed for specific training or instructional programs. To complement and increase the effectiveness of these programs, many are accompanied by printed materials such as teacher manuals, student workbooks, or scripts.

Information Services: Federal audiovisual materials are available through the following programs: *Sales*: Various audiovisual formats are available for purchase through the Center, including motion pictures, slide sets, audiotapes, and multimedia kits. Media conversion to special formats is available on request.

Preview prior to purchase is available for 16 mm motion pictures. *Rental*: Only 16 mm motion pictures, representing 80 percent of the Center's collection, are available through the rental program. *Loan Referrals*: Free loan distribution of 16 mm motion pictures is often available to the public from commercial distributors and from regional federal agency offices. The Center keeps informed of federally sponsored free loan programs and refers the user to the closest free loan source.

The Center maintains a master data file on audiovisual materials produced by the U.S. Government. This resource is used by the reference staff to respond to inquiries. There is no charge for reference service.

Printed materials issued by the Center are the principal means of keeping the public informed of the availability of federal audiovisual materials. Catalogs of listings from over 12,000 titles available for sale and/or rental are issued regularly. Also available are brochures on single and multiple titles and filmographies listing titles by subject, media, or the agency responsible for the audiovisual production. A publication entitled *Special Education* lists a wide variety of materials on early, elementary, secondary, adult, and parent education geared to persons with specific disabilities. Publications of the Center are available free upon request.

Technology Utilization Program (TU)
National Aeronautics and Space
  Administration (NASA)
600 Independence Ave., S.W.
Washington, DC 20546
(202) 755-2420

Handicapping Conditions Served: All handicaps.

The Organization: The National Aeronautics and Space Administration (NASA) Technology Utilization Program (TU), as part of its mission, adapts aerospace technology to the development of equipment for the prevention of illness and the care of the sick, handicapped, and elderly. NASA's TU Program operates in areas from bioengineering to human services delivery. Among the products that have been developed using aerospace technology are: rechargeable pacemakers; portable cassette units for electrocardiograms; coin operated high blood pressure machines; a voice controlled wheelchair which responds to 35 one-word commands; "Meals for the Homebound," food which can be easily prepared and is designed for mailing and long storage without refrigeration; a foldable walker designed for use on stairs; and a cardiology mannequin that can simulate 40 heart disease conditions with a high degree of realism for the education of medical students in cardiology.

Information Services: Information on manufacturers of technological innovations such as the ones listed above can be obtained by writing to NASA's Scientific and Technical Information Facility, P.O. Box 8756, Baltimore-Washington International Airport, Baltimore, MD 21240. Also available is a general brochure which describes many of the technical products from NASA's TU Program entitled, *Technologies for the Handicapped and the Aged. NASA Tech Briefs*, a free indexed quarterly journal utilized by rehabilitation engineers and other interested groups, describes innovations; and *NASA SP's*, a series on complex technological advances, are also available.

Other activities sponsored by the NASA TU Program are the Industrial Application Centers, which provide access to the world's largest depository of technical data; the State Technology Application Centers (STAC), which apply technology to specific needs in states; and NASA's Computer Software and Management Information Center (COSMIC), which makes selected computer programs from NASA available to engineers and researchers.

Office of Personnel Management (OPM)
Office of Affirmative Employment Programs
Office of Selective Placement Programs
1900 E Street, N.W., Room 6514
Washington, DC 20415
(202) 632-5687

Handicapping Conditions Served: All handicaps.

The Organization: The Office of Personnel Management (OPM) is the central personnel policy agency of the Federal Government.

OPM's Office of Selective Placement Programs monitors and coordinates Federal personnel regulations and policies to ensure that handicapped individuals are not adversely affected by architectural, transportation, procedural, or attitudinal barriers. A major focus is on technical assistance to agency managers and supervisors in regard to development of understanding about disabilities, job and work site modifications, and resources for obtaining rehabilitation assistance.

Information Services: OPM provides information on all aspects of employment of handicapped individuals in the Federal Government, such as: recruitment; placement; advancement; retention of employees with disabilities; and counseling for job placement through a Selective Placement Coordinator. Selective Placement Coordinators work hand-in-hand with supervisors throughout the Federal agencies to increase awareness of the capabilities of a handicapped person and techniques for accommodating such persons. Any person may request a copy of the publication, *Handbook of Selective Placement of Persons with Physical and Mental Handicaps in Federal Civil Service Employment.*

Small Business Administration (SBA)
Special Projects Division
Office of Financing
1441 L Street, N.W.
Washington, DC 20416
(202) 653-6570

Handicapping Conditions Served: All handicaps.

The Organization: The Small Business Administration (SBA) was established to encourage, assist, and protect the interests of small businesses. Financial assistance is available through Handicapped Assistance Loans to small business concerns owned, or to be owned by handicapped individuals, and to nonprofit organizations established to employ handicapped persons.

No financial assistance will be provided if funds are otherwise available from the applicant's own resources, from a private lending institution or from other Federal, state or local programs, including SBA's regular Business or Economic Opportunity Loan Programs.

SBA may guarantee up to 90 percent, not to exceed $350,000, of a loan made by a private lending institution. Direct loans by SBA are usually limited to $100,000; in unusual circumstances they may go up to $350,000. Interest rates on direct loans are 3 percent per year. Interest rates on guaranteed loans are set by the participating lending institution and must be legal and reasonable and within a maximum allowable amount which is set periodically by SBA. No direct loan can be approved if a guaranteed loan is available.

Information Services: SBA provides information about the Handicapped Assistance Loan Program to any interested individual. SBA has offices located in major cities where individuals can apply for information and other small business training. For the addresses of these offices, write to the address above.

Veterans Administration (VA)
810 Vermont Avenue, N.W.
Washington, DC 20420
(202) 393-4120

Handicapping Conditions Served: All handicaps.

The Organization: The Veterans Administration (VA) provides a wide range of benefits to those who have served in the Armed Forces, their dependents, beneficiaries of deceased veterans, and dependent children of seriously disabled veterans. Two national offices administrate programs of financial benefits and direct health care services for veterans—the **Department of Veterans Benefits** and the **Department of Medicine and Surgery**.

The **Department of Veterans Benefits** conducts an integrated program of veteran benefits. In addition to the benefits afforded all veterans, such as funds for education, on-the-job training, home loans, insurance, and benefits provided by other Federal agencies, the service-disabled veteran is entitled to special benefits and services. These include: disability compensation for injuries, diseases or disabilities incurred while on active duty in the Armed Forces; dependency allowances for wives and children of service-disabled veterans; medical care, including hospitalization, outpatient services, nursing services, and prosthetics and sensory aid services; and vocational counseling, rehabilitation, and training. Severely disabled veterans, including the blind, paraplegic, and amputees, may be entitled to specially adapted (wheelchair) homes, automobiles, or other means of conveyance.

The **Department of Medicine and Surgery** provides hospital, nursing homes, and domiciliary care, and outpatient medical and dental care to eligible veterans, through its health care system of 173 medical centers, 91 nursing home care units, 15 domiciliary care units, and 41 outpatient clinics. The Department's divisions offer medical, psychological, educational, social, and vocational services to all qualified veterans. Special rehabilitation services for the handicapped include a blindness rehabilitation program, speech and audiology rehabilitation, driver's training for the handicapped, spinal cord injury rehabilitation, and cardiopulmonary rehabilitation.

In the Department of Medicine and Surgery, the *Office of Research and Development* (R&D) administers intramural projects and programs in medical research. The Rehabilitative Engineering Research and Development Service, a part of R&D, conducts research on prosthetics, sensory aid devices, and other equipment for handicapped individuals. The *Office of Academic Affairs*, also in the Department of Medicine and Surgery, conducts an extensive health manpower education and training program.

Information Services: Information concerning benefits and services is available from VA field offices located in many cities throughout the 50 states. Each field office is staffed with benefits counselors who advise applicants and process applications for benefits. VA field offices provide assistance to veterans seeking to appeal claims decisions; this assistance is also provided by private veterans associations, some located in VA regional offices. Each state has a toll free telephone service to VA regional offices. This service provides information about benefits as well as counseling assistance to nonambulatory persons who cannot apply for benefits in person. Information about specific rehabilitation programs may be obtained from a local medical center or by contacting the *Rehabilitation Medicine Service* at the national office. Applications for medical service may be made to VA medical centers or any VA office with medical facilities. The publication, *Federal Benefits for Veterans and Dependents,* available free from all VA offices, describes benefits, services, and eligibility requirements, and lists local offices and treatment facilities by state.

Information about medical research projects sponsored by the VA is available from the **Smithsonian Science Information Exchange (SSIE)** (see separate entry for SSIE). Although SSIE is the best access point for VA research information, the R&D Information Office can conduct computerized searches on a limited basis. Many VA sponsored studies are published in private sector professional journals.

The **Office of Technology Transfer (OTT)**, located at 252 Seventh Avenue, New York, NY 10001 (212/620-6659), maintains a reference collection on rehabilitative engineering. Organized more than 30 years ago, the collection contains books, periodicals, technical reports, reprints, patents, and audiovisuals. Materials cover a wide range of subject areas—prosthetics, orthotics, communication aids, mobility aids, driving aids, artificial eye and other cosmetic restorations, wheelchairs, mobility and reading aids for the blind and partially sighted, hearing aids, and surgical implants. The collection is available for use by all individuals, but is primarily useful to the medical, allied health, and engineering professions.

OTT is a source of information on new devices and techniques developed in the VA's rehabilitation engineering programs. Its main vehicle for dissemination of new research information is the semi-annual *Bulletin of Prosthetics Research.* The Bulletin includes scientific papers, progress reports on research projects, and abstracts of recent patents and publications. Bulletins may be purchased from the Superintendent of Documents, U.S. Government Printing Office, Washington, DC 20402. OTT provides copies of reference materials or individualized letters in response to clearly stated and specific inquiries for information.

The Statistical Review and Analysis Division (202/389-2458) of the *Reports and Statistics Service* is the principal data collection office of the VA. Statistics are available on disability compensation and the type and extent of disability for veterans with both service and non-service connected handicapping conditions. While most of the statistics compiled by this office have not been published, data are readily available to requestors. Information sheets have been published on "Selected Compensation and Pension Data by State of Residence" and "Service Connected Disability Compensation Benefits." A special study on the disabled veterans of the Vietnam era is also available. The *Annual Report* of the Administrator, which may be obtained from the Reports Preparation Division (202/389-3677) includes statistical tables on the prevalence of disability among veterans.

Part Four

PROFESSIONAL AND TRADE ORGANIZATIONS

Directory of Information Resources for the Handicapped

**Academy of Dentistry for the
    Handicapped (ADH)**
1726 Champa
Suite 422
Denver, CO 80202
(303) 573-0264

Handicapping Conditions Served: All handicaps.

The Organization: The Academy of Dentistry for the Handicapped (ADH) is an organization of dentists, dental hygienists, and allied professionals. ADH provides educational services to professionals and information and referrals to handicapped persons seeking dental treatment. The organization also acts as an advocate for improved dental treatment, research, and legislation for handicapped persons. Its affiliate organization, the National Foundation of Dentistry for the Handicapped (NFDH), has 16 dental care programs for handicapped persons who attend community educational, vocational, and residential centers. Licensed dental hygienists help staff at participating centers implement a daily toothbrushing and oral hygiene program and monitor the participant's oral hygiene on a quarterly basis. In addition, the hygienists do an annual oral health assessment of each participant, help find a dentist and financing, if needed, and follow up to see that treatment is done. NFDH also has a portable dental care program to serve homebound persons. A truck with portable dental and fixed laboratory equipment and staffed by a dental assistant is available for dentist's use at the patient's bedside. The model program began serving persons in nursing homes and private residences in Denver, Colorado, in June 1979, and will be initiated in other areas of the United States. In cooperation with state dental societies, NFDH surveys dentists in its program areas who treat handicapped and homebound persons.

Information Services: Information on preventive dentistry for the handicapped is available to lay inquirers for a nominal donation. A resource list on dental care for the handicapped includes written and audiovisual materials (including materials for the blind) for lay and professional people. For the professional, ADH publishes a journal and quarterly newsletter, and it sponsors an annual continuing education course on improved dental methods and treatment for special patients. ADH maintains a referral directory of dentists who treat handicappped persons.

**Accreditation Council for Services for Mentally
    Retarded and Other Developmentally
    Disabled Persons (AC/MRDD)**
5101 Wisconsin Avenue, N.W.
Washington, DC 20016
(202) 686-5400

Handicapping Conditions Served: Mental retardation and developmental disabilities.

The Organization: Established in 1969 in association with the Joint Commission on Accreditation of Hospitals, AC/MRDD was reorganized as an independent not-for-profit corporation in 1979. The Council's sponsoring organizations include the major developmental disability advocacy groups, and it is continuing its national voluntary accreditation program, which is applicable to all agencies providing services to developmentally disabled persons. The accreditation standards and procedures previously developed by the Council will continue to be used. Workshops and consultations are offered to help agencies implement accreditation standards and prepare for accreditation survey.

Information Services: The Council responds to questions about its accreditation process, interprets its standards, and provides information concerning requirements for adequate services for developmentally disabled persons. The *Standards for Services for Developmentally Disabled Individuals* and the *Survey Questionnaire* for use with the *Standards,* which are used by agencies in evaluating their own services and used by the Council in conducting accreditation surveys, are available from the Council.

American Art Therapy Association (AATA)
428 East Baltimore Street
Baltimore, MD 21202
(301) 528-4147

Handicapping Conditions Served: All handicaps.

The Organization: The American Art Therapy Association (AATA) was established to improve the standards of art therapy training and practice, and to widen employment opportunities for art therapists. Art therapy provides the opportunity for nonverbal expression and communication. AATA approves graduate level training programs in art therapy and registers professional art therapists.

Information Services: Literature on standards of registration, a list of university training programs, and bibliographies of professional literature are free from the Association. AATA publishes a professional journal, a newsletter, and the proceedings of its annual meetings, which may be purchased by non-members. Audiovisual materials depict art therapists working with different populations, such as mentally retarded, emotionally disturbed, and elderly individuals. Professionals and students are referred to local art therapy associations and professional contacts working in specific areas of the field.

American Association for Music Therapy (AAMT)
777 Education Building
35 West 4th Street
Washington Square
New York, NY 10003
(212) 598-3491

Handicapping Conditions Served All handicaps.

The Organization: The American Association for Music Therapy approves academic programs in music therapy and certifies professional music therapists.

Information Services: Free information is available on music therapy as a career, academic program approval, and professional registration requirements. AAMT has a suggested reading list for music therapists. For university program administrators, the Association publishes standards for evaluating students within those programs. AAMT holds one or two seminars per year, where professional papers are delivered on various aspects of music therapy. A research journal and newsletter containing information about workshops, new publications in the field, job openings, and activities of AAMT are available to members.

American Association for Rehabilitation
Therapy (AART)
P.O. Box 93
North Little Rock, AR 72116
(501) 372-8861, ext. 708

Handicapping Conditions Served: All handicaps.

The Organization: The philosophy of the American Association for Rehabilitation Therapy is that rehabilitation should begin as soon as a patient enters the hospital. Members—manual arts therapists, educational therapists, recreation therapists, and rehabilitation therapists—work mostly in hospital settings under medical supervision. AART offers national and regional educational seminars devoted to these specialty areas. The association registers professionals working in these areas who meet specific educational and experience requirements.

Information Services: AART publishes informational brochures on careers and training in each of the specialty areas. It publishes the *Directory of the Registry of Medical Rehabilitation Therapists and Specialists* and two journals, the *American Archives of Rehabilitation Therapy* and *Rehabilitation Therapy*.

American Association for Respiratory Therapy (AART)
1720 Regal Row
Dallas, TX 75235
(214) 630-3540

Handicapping Conditions Served: Respiratory conditions.

The Organization: Members of the American Association for Respiratory Therapy (AART) include professionals who provide health care to victims of lung disease, such as respiratory therapists, respiratory therapy technicians, pulmonary laboratory technicians, and critical care nurses. The Association divides into several specialty sections (e.g., clinical practice, cardiopulmonary, perinatal pediatrics, critical care, etc.); and seminars and workshops are sponsored in these areas by the national and state associations. AART offers nontraditional degree programs in conjunction with a major university.

Information Services: AART provides information on professional training and career opportunities for respiratory therapists, and publishes a list of approved schools of respiratory therapy. Information is provided to professionals on diagnostic evaluation and treatment of respiratory conditions and on equipment and special devices used in respiratory therapy. The Association publishes continuing education materials for each specialty area. Monthly publications include a professional journal and a feature magazine about people working in the profession. Most information is free.

American Association of Psychiatric Services for Children (AAPSC)
1725 K Street, N.W.
Washington, DC 20006
(202) 659-9115

Handicapping Conditions Served: Mental and emotional disorders.

The Organization: The American Association of Psychiatric Services for Children (AAPSC) is a membership organization of psychiatric clinics and services and professionals specializing in the field of child mental health. The Association stresses high quality standards for clinical practice, training, and services among its goals. Towards those aims, AAPSC offers consultation to service providers on planning, development, evaluation, standards, accreditation, and financing of child mental health facilities. AAPSC supports and conducts research, represents the concerns of its membership before Congress and Federal agencies, and cooperates with other professional organizations in developing strategies to increase the impact of mental health considerations on the health planning process. A roster of available staff positions in the child mental health care field is maintained at the national office.

Information Services: AAPSC's legislative activities and projects of AAPSC members are reported in a quarterly newsletter. The Association publishes the results of its own studies (a forthcoming publication addresses professional training needs) and papers from its annual conference. At the conference, short courses are offered for continuing education credits on aspects of child mental health care. AAPSC provides referral services for emotionally disturbed children.

**American Association of University
   Affiliated Programs for the
   Developmentally Disabled**
2033 M Street, N.W., Suite 406
Washington, DC 20036
(202) 333-7880

Handicapping Conditions Served: Developmental disabilities.

The Organization: The purpose of the Association is to provide a central office and focal point to the 48 University Affiliated Facilities (UAF) located across the nation. UAFs meet the needs of developmentally disabled persons through the following services: a) comprehensive and interdisciplinary training of a broad range of professionals and para-professional persons; and b) comprehensive and interdisciplinary screening, evaluation, treatment, planning, and educational programming.

UAFs are located at or affiliated with leading colleges and universities in the country. The Association also works with HEW's agencies dealing with developmental disabilities and with congressional committees and their staffs.

Information Services: Lay and professional inquirers can request information on education and employment in professions serving developmentally disabled individuals. Also, the Association provides technical assistance for personnel dealing with developmentally disabled persons.

Publications on how to improve services for disabled individuals, and data on UAF reports on conferences are available upon request. Most publications are free of charge. Sample publications are: *The Employment Bulletin,* which includes a listing on jobs in developmental disabilities; and the *Association Newsletter,* which includes information about activities at each of the UAF centers and discussion of current issues in legislation for developmentally disabled persons.

A new UAF data base has been established in the Washington office to collect information on the 48 UAFs. Users of this data include HEW, other Federal agencies, the Association's members, and the general public.

**American Association of Workers
   for the Blind (AAWB)**
1511 K Street, N.W.
Washington, DC 20005
(202) 347-1559

Handicapping Conditions Served: Blindness and visual impairments.

The Organization: The main purpose of the American Association of Workers for the Blind (AAWB) is to provide professional enrichment through training programs and workshops for those who work with the blind. International, national, regional, and local workshops are held in 14 categories of special service to the blind, such as rehabilitation counseling, social work, reading and information services, orientation and mobility, sheltered workshops, and deaf/blind services. These workshops feature new information relevant to the specialty and successful models of service delivery. A job exchange service is provided to members of AAWB in each of the 14 specialty areas. Membership is available to anyone; most members are agencies or individuals involved in work for the blind.

Information Services: The organization operates as a clearinghouse for informational materials on aspects of blindness and on working with the blind. Most materials are free. *Blindness,* an annual collection of professional papers pertinent to working with the blind, is available from AAWB. A quarterly newsletter for members features chapter news and new developments in legislation and in work for the blind.

**American Association on Mental
    Deficiency (AAMD)**
5101 Wisconsin Avenue, N.W.
Washington, DC 20016
(202) 685-5400

Handicapping Conditions Served: Mental retardation.

The Organization: The American Association on Mental Deficiency is an organization of professionals working in the field of mental retardation established to improve services to the mentally retarded. The Association has 35 state chapters organized into 9 geographic areas and several divisions and subdivisions for specific professional disciplines. AAMD and each regional association hold annual conferences where workshops and seminars (some for continuing education credits) are offered on a variety of topics related to serving the mentally retarded.

Information Services: AAMD publishes two professional journals—*The American Journal on Mental Deficiency*, devoted to research in the field, and *Mental Retardation*, devoted to program activities for the mentally retarded. The Association's testing materials include: an *Adaptive Behavior Scale*, a test to measure the abilities of the retarded; a *Public School Version-Adaptive Behavior Scale*; and the *AAMD-Becker Reading-Free Vocational Interest Inventory*. Other publications include a *Manual on Terminology and Classification, Sociobehavioral Studies in Mental Retardation*, and AAMD official policy statements. Each region publishes its own newsletter.

**American Corrective Therapy
    Association (ACTA)**
Route 2, Elmhill
Jonesboro, TN 37659
(615) 926-1171

Handicapping Conditions Served: All handicaps.

The Organization: The American Corrective Therapy Association (ACTA) recommends standards for certification of professionals and for training facilities. It offers a limited number of scholarships to students and funds professional research. Under medical supervision, the corrective therapist adapts physical education techniques and activities to the needs of patients with specific disabilities.

Information Services: The Association is a source of information about education and training of corrective therapists. A publications list, available on request, includes titles of reprints, handbooks, and manuals on standards and practice in the field. These publications are available at a minimal charge. ACTA publishes a professional journal which is clinical and research oriented. The Executive Director, Mr. Kirk Hodges, may be contacted at his work number (listed above) or by mail.

American Dance Therapy Association (ADTA)
2000 Century Plaza
Suite 230
Columbia, MD 21044
(301) 997-4040

Handicapping Conditions Served: All handicaps.

The Organization: The American Dance Therapy Association (ADTA) approves educational programs in dance therapy and registers professional dance therapists.

Information Services: ADTA has free information on educational programs, guidelines for dance therapy training and internship, professional registration requirements, and regional professional contacts. The Association publishes *The American Journal of Dance Therapy* (available at reduced rates to members), a newsletter, monographs, bibliographies and reports of conference proceedings which are free to members and are available for a charge to nonmembers. ADTA sponsors annual educational workshops, and its regional chapters hold similar workshops throughout the year. Nonmembers are welcome to attend.

American Deafness and Rehabilitation
Association (ADARA)
814 Thayer Avenue
Silver Spring, MD 20910
(301) 589-0880 (Voice or TTY)

Handicapping Conditions Served: Deafness and hearing impairments.

The Organization: The American Deafness and Rehabilitation Association offers a forum for the exchange of information to professionals who work with the deaf, such as rehabilitation personnel, interpreters, speech and hearing therapists, physicians, and psychologists. Mainly through its literature, ADARA emphasizes the unique rehabilitation needs of the deaf adult. The Association has three special interest sections of counselors, state deaf-blind coordinators and state rehabilitation coordinators, whose members exchange information through correspondence and meetings. There are five state chapters of ADARA. The organization was formerly known as Professional Rehabilitation Workers with the Adult Deaf (PRWAD).

Information Services: A quarterly professional journal contains articles related to new techniques, innovative programs or practices, and research relevant to rehabilitation. ADARA's monthly newsletter reports on activities of the organization and its chapters, and includes special interest sections and lists of job openings in various fields of work with the deaf. The national office can provide general information on careers (university programs and employment settings) and referrals to professionals in specific fields of work with deaf adults.

American Library Association (ALA)
Association of Specialized and
Cooperative Library Agencies (ASCLA)
50 East Huron Street
Chicago, IL 60611
(312) 944-6780

Handicapping Conditions Served: All handicaps.

The Organization: The Association of Specialized and Cooperative Library Agencies, a division of the American Library Association, is a professional organization for librarians serving communities and special populations such as the blind, physically handicapped, deaf, and impaired elderly. ASCLA serves in an advisory capacity, helping its members to develop and evaluate policies and activities.

Information Services: Standards and guidelines for libraries developing services for the blind and mentally retarded are available in print form. Special issues of the ASCLA journal which relate to library services to the handicapped are: *Bibliotherapy, Information Needs of Hearing Impaired People*, and *Library Services for the Blind and Physically Handicapped*. Other publications available from ALA or ASCLA include *The Librarian and the Patient, The Special Child in the Library*, and *Equal Access: A Manual of Procedures for Initiating a Public Library Home Service Program*. ASCLA publishes a quarterly newsletter and members issue a periodic newsletter on service to the developmentally disabled. For additional information, contact Sandra M. Cooper, Executive Secretary, ASCLA.

**American Occupational Therapy
  Association (AOTA)**
6000 Executive Boulevard
Rockville, MD 20852
(301) 770-2200

Handicapping Conditions Served: All handicaps and the aged.

The Organization: The American Occupational Therapy Association (AOTA) promotes quality occupational therapy (OT) services by providing accreditation of educational programs, certification of practitioners, professional development, public education, and advocacy on programs related to national health care issues.

Information Services: Information is available to the general public about OT as a career and schools that offer professional programs in OT. A variety of print and audiovisual materials for the OT practitioner are published and sold by the organization. AOTA has free professional information packets on 15 subject areas including arthritis, alcoholism, cerebral palsy, geriatrics, and spinal cord injuries. These packets contain the names of OT resource persons who specialize in the particular field, special facilities, bibliographies of printed materials, and selected reprints. The Association sponsors regional workshops on such topics as sensory integration, prosthetics, orthotics, OT and pediatrics, and reality orientation for the elderly. AOTA publishes a monthly professional journal, a monthly newsletter, and a *Federal Report,* available by subscription. The organization's state associations provide inquirers with referrals to local OT practitioners and facilities.

**American Orthotic and Prosthetic
  Association (AOPA)**
1440 N Street, N.W.
Washington, DC 20005
(202) 234-8400

Handicapping Conditions Served: Musculoskeletal and orthopedic conditions.

The Organization: The American Orthotic and Prosthetic Association (AOPA) represents the interests of manufacturers and retailers of orthotic and prosthetic devices by interacting with government agencies and assisting in preparation of Federal and state legislation. National and regional meetings are held to keep members of the profession abreast of technological advances and to discuss facility management.

Information Services: A list of training facilities for students interested in entering the orthotics and prosthetics field is available from the Association. AOPA publishes a journal and a news magazine which emphasize professional, technical, and business topics. A listing of members is compiled annually. AOPA has written a *Medicare Manual* to assist professionals in obtaining Medicare payments. Publications are free to members and available to nonmembers for purchase. For additional information, contact Sonja McCamley, Assistant Executive Director.

**American Physical Therapy
  Association (APTA)**
1156 15th Street, N.W.
Washington, DC 20005
(202) 466-2070

Handicapping Conditions Served: All physical handicaps and mental retardation.

The Organization: The American Physical Therapy Association (APTA) fosters the development and improvement of physical therapy services and education by: 1) accrediting academic programs in physical therapy; 2) assisting in composing state certification examinations; and 3) offering continuing education courses and workshops in specialty areas (e.g., arthritis, central nervous system disorders, burn treatment, sports medicine, etc.) at the national and local level. For its members, APTA provides research felllowships and legal assistance for alleged malpractice. APTA operates a job bank for members and nonmembers.

Information Services: Free information is available about physical therapy as a career, opportunities for minorities in the field, accredited professional training programs, sources of financial assistance for students, and employment statistics. A free pamphlet is available on the prevention of joggging injuries, back pain, and stiffness due to degenerative arthritis. APTA publishes a professional journal and a newsletter as well as books related to practice in the field. A publications list is available. APTA refers handicapped individuals to facilities which offer physical therapy services and to sources for obtaining prosthetic aids (manufacturers, catalogs, or retail outlets). For further information, contact Phyllis Quinn, Director of Information Central.

**American Speech-Language-Hearing
   Association (ASHA)**
10801 Rockville Pike
Rockville, MD 20852
(301) 897-5700

Handicapping Conditions Served: Speech, language, and hearing disorders.

The Organization: The American Speech-Language-Hearing Association (ASHA) is a certifying body for professionals providing speech, language, and hearing therapy to the public, and is an accrediting agency for college and university graduate school programs in speech-language pathology and audiology, and for clinic and hospital programs which offer such services. The Association conducts research in communication disorders and studies of community needs for direct services.

Information Services: Public information brochures about communication disorders and the roles of professional therapists are available from ASHA. ASHA has extensive career information in the areas of possible employment, university training programs, and certification requirements. Its publications include the *Journal of Speech and Hearing Research; Journal of Speech and Hearing Disorders; Language, Speech and Hearing Services in the Schools; Guide to Clinical Services in Speech-Language Pathology and Audiology; Guide to Graduate Education in Speech-Language Pathology and Audiology;* and an *ASHA Directory* of membership. A monthly magazine, *Asha*, features organizational news, announcements of meetings, job openings, and research reports. Some publications are free to members, but all may be subscribed to or purchased by interested persons. Forty-seven state affiliates provide information about clinical services at the local level, and some publish their own newsletters. ASHA sponsors conferences, short courses, institutes, and workshops as part of its professional education program.

**Association for Education of the
   Visually Handicapped (AEVH)**
919 Walnut Street
Fourth Floor
Philadelphia, PA 19107
(215) 923-7555

Handicapping Conditions Served: Blindness, visual impairments, and deaf-blindness.

The Organization: The Association for Education of the Visually Handicapped (AEVH) is a membership organization of teachers and others who work with blind and visually impaired children. AEVH establishes professional standards and certifies teachers and paraprofessionals working in the field. Special interest groups of AEVH, including house parents, itinerant and resource teachers, teachers of the multihandicapped and deaf-blind, and orientation and mobility instructors, meet annually to conduct educational workshops in their specialized fields.

Information Services: The Association publishes a professional journal, a newsletter, and papers from its educational workshops. *Working with Visually Handicapped Persons* presents career and college information for prospective teachers and paraprofessionals.

Association of Medical Rehabilitation Directors and Coordinators (AMRDC)
3830 Linklea Drive
Houston, TX 77025
(713) 665-4253

Handicapping Conditions Served: All handicaps.

The Organization: Members of the Association are physicians in rehabilitation medicine and directors or coordinatiors of rehabilitation programs. The organization sets standards for professional practice, and provides professional certification to qualifying members. It offers continuing education courses in rehabilitation management in conjunction with its annual meeting, and it provides a job placement service for members.

Information Services: Information about professional certification and university programs in rehabilitation management is available from the Association. AMRDC publishes an annual membership directory and a quarterly newsletter, which covers Association activities and reviews publications relevant to the field.

Association of Mental Health Administrators (AMHA)
The Pennsylvania Building
Suite 1230
425 13th Street, N.W.
Washington, DC 20004
(202) 638-6662

Handicapping Conditions Serves: Mental and emotional disorders and developmental disabilities.

The Organization: The purpose of the Association of Mental Health Administrators (AMHA) is to improve administration in the mental health field. To that end, AMHA establishes accreditation and certification standards for the profession and offers continuing education programs. The Association operates a telephone consulting network, whereby inquirers may contact experienced administrators who specialize in specific areas. AMHA has a free job placement service for its members.

Information Services: AMHA and its 20 chapters sponsor year-round regional and state seminars and workshops for managers at all levels of administration. Topics include: 1) deinstitutionalizing mentally retarded persons; 2) milieus for the multihandicapped; 3) accreditation of facilities; and 4) improving community relations. Queries about federal rules, regulations, and requirements for mental health facilities are answered by phone or by mail. AMHA's membership newsletter covers chapter activities, legislative news, job openings and employee availabilities, and summaries of relevant publications.

**Association on Handicapped Student
Service Programs in Post-Secondary
Education (AHSSPPE)**
Box 8256 University Station
Grand Forks, ND 58202
(701) 777-3425

Handicapping Conditions Served: All handicaps.

The Organization: The Association on Handicapped Student Services Programs in Post-Secondary Education (AHSSPPE) provides a vehicle to strengthen the professionalism, expertise, and competence of personnel working with post-secondary handicapped students.

The Association was established on March 4, 1978, and members represent residential and non-residential campuses, two-year and four-year/graduate level institutions. The Association has sponsored several workshops and conferences.

Information Services: The Association publishes a newsletter, *ALERT*, which is distributed to members. Membership is open to all interested persons.

Better Hearing Institute (BHI)
1430 K Street, N.W., Suite 600
Washington, DC 20005
(202) 638-7577
(800) 424-8576

Handicapping Conditions Served: Hearing impairments.

The Organization: The Better Hearing Institute (BHI) serves the hearing impaired through public information and public service programs, informing them about hearing loss and readily available medical, surgical, hearing aid, and rehabilitation assistance.

Information Services: BHI produces an extensive series of public service announcements on radio and TV, which often feature various celebrities with corrected hearing handicaps. The Institute also produces booklets, articles, and slide-tape presentations on hearing loss and what to do about it, which BHI sells to community organizations. Examples of the slide/cassette programs are: "You and Your Hearing," for general audiences; "Silence Is Lonely," targeted to the special needs of the senior citizen; and "We Overcame Hearing Loss," narrated by comedian Norm Crosby. Sample speeches and printed materials on hearing loss, including noise-induced hearing loss, are also available from BHI. There is a charge for printed and audiovisual materials.

A Hearing HelpLine, (800) 424-8576, provides assistance to professionals, law enforcement officials, and consumers in handling questions, suggestions and complaints about hearing loss, hearing aids, and hearing aid services. BHI has national listings of speech and hearing clinics, otolaryngologists, and certified hearing aid dispensers. Information from Hearing HelpLine is free.

**Commission on Accreditation of
Rehabilitation Facilities (CARF)**
2500 North Pantano Road
Tucson, AZ 85715
(602) 886-8575

Handicapping Conditions Served: All handicaps.

The Organization: The Commission on Accreditation of Rehabilitation Facilities (CARF) establishes standards for and accredits rehabilitation facilities involved in physical restoration, personal and social adjustment, vocational development, sheltered employment, work activity, speech pathology, and audiology.

Information Services: Basic information about standards affecting all aspects of a rehabilitation facility's operation may be obtained from CARF's *Standards Manual for Rehabilitation Facilities.* The Commission publishes separate pamphlets on program evaluation for specific facilities: hospital based facilities, vocational rehabilitation centers, work activity centers, and outpatient rehabilitation facilities. A self-study questionnaire is free to facilities wishing to conduct self-evaluations before CARF's on-site visit. A list of accredited facilities is available upon request. For additiona information, contact Jack L. Nichols, Associate Director.

Conference of Executives of American
Schools for the Deaf (CEASD)
5034 Wisconsin Avenue, N.W.
Washington, DC 20016
(202) 363-1327

Handicapping Conditions Served: Deafness, hearing impairments, and deaf-blindness.

The Organization: The Conference of Executives of American Schools for the Deaf (CEASD) was founded to promote effective management of schools, programs, and agencies providing services to the deaf. Its standing committees have developed position papers on topics related to the administration of elementary, secondary, postsecondary, and residential schools for the deaf. Administrative workshops are held throughout the year on these topics. CEASD evaluates and accredits elementary and secondary school programs, and certifies individuals who work in residential settings.

Information Services: The CEASD Captioned Films Distribution Center, sponsored by grants from the Department of Health, Education, and Welfare, selects and distributes captioned educational films and distributes captioned general entertainment films. These films are available on loan to deaf groups.

The Conference and the Convention of American Instructors of the Deaf jointly publish the *American Annals of the Deaf,* which includes a variety of articles relevant to the deaf and to professionals working with the deaf. Each April issue of the *Annals* is a *Directory of Programs and Services for the Deaf in the United States,* listing local educational and rehabilitative services for the deaf, including the deaf-blind, in the U.S. and Canada. CEASD publishes the proceedings of its annual conference and copies of its administrative position papers. Members receive a newsletter. An extensive materials list of pamphlets and reprints from the *Annals* is available from the Conference.

Convention of American Instructors
of the Deaf (CAID)
5034 Wisconsin Avenue, N.W.
Washington, DC 20016
(202) 363-1327

Handicapping conditions Served: Deafness, hearing impairments, and deaf-blindness.

The Organization: Members of the Convention of American Instructors of the Deaf (CAID) include teachers and support personnel working in a variety of educational settings. Through biennial conferences and regional workshops, CAID promotes the exchange of information among professionals. Topics for workshops range from diagnostic tools to sex education to psycholinguistics. Through its membership in the Council of Education of the Deaf, CAID helps to formulate standards of professional certification and accreditation of educational programs.

Information Services: CAID and the Conference of Executives of American Schools for the Deaf jointly publish the *American Annals of the Deaf,* which includes a variety of articles relevant to the deaf and to professionals working with the deaf. Each April issue of the *Annals* is a *Directory of Programs and Services for the Deaf in the United States,* listing local educational and rehabilitative services for the deaf, including the deaf-blind, in the U.S. and Canada. Reprints from the *Annals* and a materials list containing pamphlets of interest to teachers, students, and parents are available from CAID. The organization publishes a newsletter for members and proceedings from its conferences.

**Council of State Administrators of
    Vocational Rehabilitation (CSAVR)**
1522 K Street, N.W.
Suite 610
Washington, DC 20005
(202) 638-4634

Handicapping Conditions Served: All handicaps.

The Organization: The Council of State Administrators of Vocational Rehabilitation (CSAVR) is composed of the chief administrators of vocational rehabilitation agencies in the states, the District of Columbia, and the four U.S. territories. These agencies serve physically and mentally handicapped persons and are the state partners in the Federal-state program of vocational rehabilitation services provided under the Rehabilitation Act of 1973. In addition to providing a forum for discussion of relevant issues to its member administrators, the Council serves as an advisory body to the Rehabilitation Services Administration, HEW, and the National Rehabilitation Association.

Information Services: CSAVR provides information to member agencies and to Federal agencies in coordinating vocational rehabilitation services.

Deafness Research Foundation (DRF)
342 Madison Avenue
New York, NY 10017
(212) 682-3737

Handicapping Conditions Served: Deafness and hearing impairments.

The Organization: The Deafness Research Foundation (DRF) was founded in 1958 to find support for new research into the causes, treatment, and prevention of deafness. DRF provides seed grants for ear research projects at hospitals, research laboratories, and universities in the U.S. and Canada. The Centurions of the DFR, an organization of physicians, audiologists, and researchers, contributes its membership dues to meet the basic administrative expenses of the DRF, thus making it possible for all public contributions to go directly into the funding of ear research.

With the endorsement of the American Academy of Otolaryngology and the National Association of the Deaf, the DRF sponsors the **National Temporal Bone Banks Program (NTBB)** and seeks individual pledges of temporal bones to be used for research and physician training.

Information Services: DRF publishes two periodic newsletters: a technical research publication for members of the Centurions; and a lay publication, *The Receiver,* which reports current research and provides practical tips for dealing with specific ear diseases and hearing problems. A third newsletter is planned for temporal bone donors.

DRF makes referrals to medical centers, medical specialists, audiology centers, and voluntary agencies concerned with deafness and hearing impairments. Information about NTBB may be obtained from DRF or NTBB regional centers located in Boston, Minneapolis, Houston, and Los Angeles.

**Foundation for Science
and the Handicapped**
56788 Meadowood Drive
Elkhart, IN 46514
(219) 264-8746

Handicapping Conditions Served: All handicaps.

The Organization: The Foundation for Science and the Handicapped was established in 1977 by a group of disabled scientists. The Foundation seeks to improve the quality and accessibility of the educational system for handicapped individuals. Major goals are to build a network that will support handicapped scientists throughout their lives, and involve Foundation members in advisory committees in academe, government, and industry. The Foundation works closely with the American Association for the Advancement of Science.

Information Services: Membership information can be obtained from the membership chairman, Mr. Louis G. Dannora, at the above address. Any handicapped individual who is interested in a science career can contact the Foundation for information.

**National Accreditation Council for Agencies
Serving the Blind and Visually
Handicapped (NAC)**
79 Madison Avenue, Suite 1406
New York, NY 10016
(212) 683-8581

Handicapping Conditions Served: Blindness and visual impairments.

The Organization: The National Accreditation Council for Agencies Serving the Blind and Visually Handicapped (NAC) establishes and maintains accreditation standards for agencies and schools that specialize in serving blind children and adults. The Council accredits such organizations that meet its standards and reviews services and management periodically to assure continued worthiness for accredited status.

Information Services: NAC provides information about its standards which are published in the form of self-study and evaluation guides. Guides are presently available for 23 types of services which fall into the basic categories of management functions and the services of agencies and specialized schools. Publication descriptions and an order form list the specific guides which may be purchased for a nominal fee. Free publications include a current list of accredited members, a fact sheet on consumer rights, a newsletter, and an annual report. These are available in inkprint and on flexible disc sound recordings. The guides and other publications may be obtained in tape recorded form and in large print via microfiche. For more information, contact Carl Augusto, Assistant Director, or Dr. Richard Bleecker, Executive Director.

**National Association for
Music Therapy (NAMT)**
901 Kentucky, Suite 206
P.O. Box 610
Lawrence, KS 66044
(913) 842-1909

Handicapping Conditions Served: All handicaps.

The Organization: The National Association for Music Therapy (NAMT) promotes the development of music as therapy by: 1) approving university curricula for music therapy programs; 2) approving clinical facilities for training music therapists; 3) certifying and registering professional music therapists; and 4) providing informational assistance to researchers in the field of music therapy.

Information Services: Free publications of NAMT include brochures about music therapy as a career (both for the prospective student and the career counselor), a yearly guide to conferences and workshops across the country, and an audiovisual catalog. Other publications of the Association, such as *Music Therapy Clinical Training Facilities Handbook* and *Handbook for Volunteer Workers in Hospital Music,* are sold. A quarterly journal that contains reports of original investigations and theoretical papers pertaining to music therapy is free to members; subscriptions are sold to nonmembers. Additional membership materials may also be purchased by nonmembers. Handicapped inquirers are referred to music therapists or to facilities which employ music therapists. For information, contact Mrs. Margaret S. Sears, Executive Director, at the above address.

National Association of Private
Residential Facilities for the
Mentally Retarded (NAPRFMR)
6269 Leesburg Pike, Suite B-5
Falls Church, VA 22044
(703) 536-3311

Handicapping Conditions Served: Mental retardation, cerebral palsy, autism, epilepsy, and other developmental disabilities.

The Organization: The National Association of Private Residential Facilities for the Mentally Retarded (NAPRFMR) was founded in 1970 to improve the quality of life for developmentally disabled persons and their families by coordinating the efforts of providers of private residential services. Active membership is open to any state or locally approved facility or home serving primarily developmentally disabled persons. Associate membership is available to any interested person, organization, or facility not qualifying for active membership.

The Association offers comprehensive insurance protection for member facilities.

Information Services: NAPRFMR conducts conferences and studies, and issues bulletins and a newsletter to keep its members informed of current legislation and regulations, safety and access standards, funding sources, social security benefits, the rights of disabled persons and their parents, staff development techniques, and topics of current interest. The newsletter is free to members. A *Directory of Members,* which lists facilities by state, is available at $15.

NAPRFMR responds to inquiries from members and the public. Information is strong in the areas of placement for developmentally disabled persons and government activities of interest to private operators of residential facilities.

National Association of Private Schools
for Exceptional Children (NAPSEC)
130 East Orange Avenue
Lake Wales, FL 33853
(813) 676-2250

Handicapping Conditions Served: All handicaps.

The Organization: The Association acts as an approving body for private schools which serve the handicapped and as a communication link among member shcools and between the members and local, state and Federal agencies.

Information Services: NAPSEC publishes a directory of members which describes services offered and populations served. A *Guide to Special Education and Federal Law* and information about requirements and procedures for approval are also available. A newsletter is published three times a year and is distributed free to individuals, institutions, agencies, and associations.

National Association of Rehabilitation
   Facilities (NARF)
5530 Wisconsin Avenue
Suite 955
Washington, DC 20015
(301) 654-5882

Handicapping Conditions Served: All handicaps.

The Organization: The National Association of Rehabilitation Facilities (NARF) was formed by a merger of the Association of Rehabilitation Centers and the National Association of Sheltered Workshops and Homebound Programs. Its membership is made up of institutions and individuals that offer rehabilitation services. The purpose of the Association is to strengthen rehabilitation services to the handicapped by representing the interests of these services to the Federal Government, and by offering management training seminars to professionals. Twenty-one state chapters work to improve facilities at the state and local levels, through various representative committees (e.g. committees on vocational facilities, medical facilities, developmental centers. etc.).

Information Services: NARF has information about federal legislation affecting rehabilitation facilities. Although the national Association refers handicapped persons to facilities (educational, vocational, and medical), state chapters tend to have more complete local listings. NARF 3-day training seminars are held in various locations at all times of the year on subjects related to the management and operation of rehabilitation facilities. NARF publishes periodicals, bulletins, and newsletters for rehabilitation service administrators, including funding information for rehabilitation programs.

National Association of State Directors
   of Special Education (NASDSE)
1201 Sixteenth Street, N.W.
Washington, DC 20036
(202) 833-4218

Handicapping Conditions Served: All handicaps.

The Organization: The National Association of State Directors of Special Education (NASDSE) is a nonprofit association representing personnel from state education agencies who have legal responsibility for the administration and supervision of special education programs in public schools.

Information Services: NASDSE has developed numerous products and conferences interpreting Section 504 of the Rehabilitation Act and Public Law 94-142, the Education for All Handicapped Children Act. Most products are sold as training packages for state directors and local level personnel interested in federal programs affecting handicapped children. Twenty-five publications that include resources for workshops on awareness, information on legislation, and implementation of legislation for the handicapped are available to educational administrators. Audiovisual materials for teachers and administrators on the subject of the Individualized Education Plan (IEP) are also for sale. Twenty-six issues of the *Liaison Bulletin* are published annually, covering timely information affecting handicapped children, issues on legislation, and job opportunities in education for the handicapped. For a current brochure on products and prices write to the above address.

**National Association of State Mental
  Retardation Program Directors, Inc.
  (NASMRPD)**
20001 Jefferson Davis Highway
Suite 806
Arlington, VA 22202
(703) 920-0700

Handicapping Conditions Served: Mental retardation and developmental disabilities.

The Organization: The organization's membership consists of 53 state mental retardation (MR) program directors. NASMRPD facilitates the exchange of information among members on effective methods of providing care and treatment for the mentally retarded, and it represents the views of its members before Congress and Federal agencies.

Information Services: NASMRPD collects information about available services and model service programs for the mentally retarded and developmentally disabled (DD) in each state. Areas of information include education, employment programs, public and private residential programs, foster care, early diagnosis and screening programs, recreation, and staff training programs. NASMRPD has Federal and state legislative information in all areas affecting the MR field, including health, education, welfare, Social Security, housing, employment, and transportation issues. Anyone may request information, but because of staff limitations, priority is given to members' requests. The Association publishes two monthly newsletters, one focusing on innovative state programs, *New Directions*; the other on legislative developments affecting the mentally retarded, *Capitol Capsule*. It also publishes special reports analyzing legislation related to the MR/DD population. National and regional meetings, featuring seminars on specific service-need categories, are held primarily for directors and staff of state MR programs, but anyone may attend.

**National Association of Vocational Education
  Special Needs Personnel (NAVESNP)**
American Vocational Association (AVA)
2020 North 14th Street
Arlington, VA 22201
(703) 522-6121

Handicapping Conditions Served: All handicaps.

The Organization: The National Association of Vocational Education Special Needs Personnel (NAVESNP) is a membership segment of the American Vocational Association (AVA) devoted to personnel working with handicapped and disadvantaged youth. Members include special needs personnel, vocational counselors, and vocational education and special education teachers, working at the secondary and postsecondary levels. NAVESNP attempts to provide improved services to special populations by acting as a communication network and information center for professionals working with such populations.

Information Services: NAVESNP publishes a professional journal and a newsletter (containing information on meetings, tips for teachers, and Federal legislation) three times a year; a directory of teachers; and other publications which relate to vocational education and the handicapped.

NAVESNP holds regional workshops throughout the year. Topics range from jobs and careers for the handicapped to teaching vocational reading and mathematics. While these workshops are mainly for professional education, parents of handicapped children are welcome to attend.

**National Council for Homemaker-Home Health
Aide Services**
67 Irving Place
New York, NY 10003
(212) 674-4990

Handicapping Conditions Served: All handicaps.

The Organization: The goal of the National Council is to bring health and homemaker services to families whose homes have been disrupted by illness, disability, emotional, and other problems. In all sections of the nation, in-the-home services are needed to help individuals and families in all economic brackets. To make these services available, the Council evaluates local agencies for accreditation, and encourages the formation of new services through a Federal and state advocacy project. It provides technical assistance to new agencies, and offers training workshops at the state level to administrators, supervisors, and aides.

Information Services: The Council has an extensive publications list of print and audiovisual materials relevant to the consumer needing homemaker-health aide services and the professional delivering those services. The organization's professional materials are particularly strong in the areas of establishing programs, training professionals, and providing services to particular populations (e.g. the elderly, children, mentally retarded, terminally ill, etc.). The Council prepares two service directories: one, a comprehensive list of services in the U.S., Puerto Rico, and the Virgin Islands; and the second, a list of those services which are accredited by the Council. The Council operates a lending library, free to member agencies but with a nominal charge to nonmembers. For additional information, contact Mr. Leslie L. Clark, Director of Communications.

**National Council for Therapy and
Rehabilitation through Horticulture
(NCTRH)**
Mount Vernon, VA 22121
(703) 836-3306

Handicapping Conditions Served: All handicaps.

The Organization: The National Council for Therapy and Rehabilitation through Horticulture (NCTRH) acts as a consultant to institutions interested in establishing horticulture therapy programs. It also registers professional horticulture therapists and sponsors regional professional workshops in conjunction with its six state chapters and with university programs. NCTRH operates a job bank for members and nonmembers.

Information Services: Information is available on careers in horticultural therapy. Special publications are printed periodically to offer a means of continuing education to professionals on such topics as innovative programs and funding sources. NCTRH has bibliographic and audiovisual materials for persons to use in the field or to start a program. It also maintains a speakers' bureau. Members receive a monthly newsletter.

National Education Association (NEA)
1201 16th Street, N.W.
Washington, DC 20036
(202) 833-4000

Handicapping Conditions Served: All handicaps.

The Organization: The NEA is a professional organization of elementary and secondary school teachers, administrators, principals, and counselors. NEA's involvement with handicapped students' concerns is in the area of the Education for All Handicapped Children Act (Public Law 94-142).

Information Services: The NEA informs its members about the law and its implications for them and their students; gathers teacher testimony about the effects of the law in order to bring about changes in the law; informs teachers of their legal rights in matters pertaining to P.L. 94-142 and handles grievances or suits that occur; and lobbies for increased funding for that Act. Members may obtain *A Teacher's Reference Guide to P.L. 94-142* and reprints of articles on disabilities and how they affect the educational process.

National Eye Research Foundation (NERF)
18 South Michigan Avenue
Chicago, IL 60603
(312) 726-7866

Handicapping Conditions Served: Blindness and visual impairments.

The Organization: The National Eye Research Foundation is a membership organization for ophthalmologists, opticians, and other professional and lay people interested in the eye care field. With the objective of improving eye care for the general public, it sponsors research projects in the field of ophthalmology, and disseminates research information on practical innovations and techniques to professionals. Dissemination is through international, national, and regional meetings, and through public service announcements.

Information Services: For lay inquirers, NERF provides free brochures defining specialties within the eye care profession and defining certain eye disorders, such as glaucoma, hyperopia, and myopia. The organization makes referrals to local eye specialists. NERF's bimonthly research journal on contact lenses, *Contacto*, is available to members only. For further information, contact Mrs. Waneta Reynolds, Coordinating Secretary.

National Hearing Aid Society (NHAS)
20361 Middlebelt Road
Livonia, MI 48152
(313) 478-2610
(800) 521-5248

Handicapping Conditions Served: Deafness and hearing impairments.

The Organization: The National Hearing Aid Society (NHAS) establishes training and ethical standards for professionals who fit and sell hearing aids. Its certification process outlines the educational, experience, and ethical requirements needed to become a Certified Hearing Aid Audiologist. NHAS offers an independent, self-paced study course in hearing aid audiology. Other training courses are reviewed by NHAS for suitability of course content. The Society acts as an intermediary between consumers and hearing aid specialists when consumers have problems with hearing aid transactions.

Information Services: A Hearing Aid Helpline, (800) 521-5247, has been established for consumers to receive basic information on hearing aid care and maintenance or assistance in resolving hearing aid transaction problems. A free consumer packet includes a directory of certified member services and a Better Business Bureau booklet, *Facts about Hearing Aids*. Other general information pamphlets about hearing loss and hearing aids are available to the consumer. For the hearing health professional, NHAS publishes a quarterly educational and research journal, a directory of member services, and several pamphlets about standards of ethics, certification, and technical information. The national Society and its 50 chapters sponsor educational workshops for professionals on subjects such as fitting techniques, acoustics, hearing testing, and ear molds.

National Rehabilitation Association (NRA)
1522 K Street, N.W.
Suite 1120
Washington, DC 20005
(202) 659-2430

Handicapping Conditions Served: All handicaps.

The Organization: The National Rehabilitation Association (NRA) was founded in 1925 as a membership organization for professionals and consumers interested in the advancement of rehabilitation services to all handicapped persons. NRA's activities include: advocacy for state and federal legislation; professional development through regular meetings and workshops, training sessions for continuing education credits, publications, and fellowships to students; and public education via print and electronic media. The NRA has 50 state chapters and seven divisions, which devote their efforts to disseminating information to professionals working in specific rehabilitation fields.

The **National Rehabilitation Counseling Association (NRCA)** is the largest NRA division and the only one with a paid staff. It is one of the sponsors of the Commission on Rehabilitation Counselor Certification. NRCA holds continuing education programs, publishes professional literature, and has a scholarship program for students in graduate rehabilitation counseling programs.

Other divisions include the Job Placement Division (JPD), National Association for Independent Living (NAIL), National Association of Rehabilitation Instructors (NARI), National Association of Rehabilitation Secretaries (NARS), National Rehabilitation Administration Association (NRAA), and the Vocational Evaluation and Work Adjustment Association (VEWAA).

Information Services: NRA publishes the *Journal of Rehabilitation* and a newsletter. The national office responds to general inquiries and directs specific questions to appropriate professional divisions.

NRCA publishes the *Journal of Applied Rehabilitation Counseling,* reports, and newsletters. NCRA may be contacted directly at Suite 1110, 1522 K Street, N.W., Washington, DC 20005, (202) 296-6080.

All the divisions publish newsletters, and RNAA publishes two quarterly journals: the *Journal of Rehabilitation Administration* and *Administration and Supervision in Rehabilitation.* The national NRA office should be contacted for the current addresses of its division officers.

National Therapeutic Recreation
Society (NTRS)
1601 N. Kent Street
Arlington, VA 22209
(703) 525-0606

Handicapping Conditions Served: All handicaps.

The Organization: The National Therapeutic Recreation Society is a membership organization for therapists who provide recreation activities to the ill, handicapped, and institutionalized in direct care facilities and in the community. NTRS is a branch of the National Recreation and Park Association (NRPA). The Society accredits recreational programs offered by colleges and universities, and acts as a professional licensing agency for recreational therapists. It offers consulting services to agencies, institutions, and individuals on new management techniques in the field.

Information Services: NRPA publishes books and brochures for the recreational therapist on providing services to specific populations. Titles include *Recreation for Disabled Children* and *Recreation in Nursing Homes.* NRPA sponsors regional and national conferences where special workshops are held for the recreational therapist on such topics as program design, facility design, and rehabilitation of special populations. A professional journal and a newsletter are available to members.

Project Heath
American Council on Education
One Dupont Circle, N.W.
Washington, DC 20036
(202) 833-4660

Handicapping Conditions Served: All handicaps.

The Organization: The American Council on Education is an umbrella organization of professional organizations in higher education. Project HEATH—Higher Education and the Handicapped—funded by the Bureau of Education for the Handicapped, the W. K. Kellogg Foundation, and a contract from the Office for Civil Rights, HEW, is a united effort of 23 major national higher education associations and consumer organizations of handicapped persons to assist the higher education community to respond creatively and constructively to the Federal requirements mandating equal access to postsecondary institutions for qualified students and employees. Six organizations play distinctive roles.

Information Services:

The American Association of Higher Education (AAHE)
One Dupont Circle, N.W.
Washington, DC 20036
(202) 293-6447 (Hotline)

Operates the HEATH Resource Center where a hotline is available Tuesday, Wednesday, and Friday, 1-5 p.m. EST to answer questions related to 504 compliance by colleges or to refer to other sources. The Center operates a clearinghouse in locating information about programs, resources, publications, training materials, and skilled personnel. The Center refers handicapped individuals to campuses where others with similar disabilities have been accommodated.

Association of Physical Plant Administrators (APPA)
11 Dupont Circle, N.W., Suite 250
Washington, DC 20036
(202) 234-1662

APPA offers technical assistance mainly for physical access questions through a hotline, (202) 234-1664. Several publications are available as well as a poster and accessibility information flyer.

American Association of Collegiate Registrars
and Admissions Officers (AACRAO)
One Dupont Circle, N.W., Suite 330
Washington, DC 20036
(202) 293-9161

AACRAO published a *Guide to Recruitment and Admission* (available free) and connects with Admission Officers who are trained and experienced in providing consultation on recruitment and admission of disabled students.

College and University Personnel Association (CUPA)
11 Dupont Circle, N.W., Suite 120
Washington, DC 20036
(202) 462-1038

CUPA trained a Technical Assistance Corps (TAC) which is now available for access questions.

American Association of Colleges of Teacher
    Education (AACTE)
One Dupont Circle, N.W., Suite 610
Washington, DC 20036
(202) 293-2450

AACTE conducts workshops on improving the role of institutions in training teachers for the education of handicapped individuals, and responds to inquiries on this subject. AACTE wants input from teachers of handicapped youth on problems they encountered and solutions they found, and invites handicapped teachers to share their experiences about barriers they encountered in getting their education and jobs.

National Association of Colleges and University
    Business Officers (NABUCO)
One Dupont Circle, N.W., Suite 510
Washington, DC 20036
(202) 296-2344

NABUCO published the *Guide to Self Evaluation for Colleges and Universities* (available free) and numerous reports and articles on access issues in the *Business Officer*.

Project on the Handicapped in Science
American Association for the Advancement of Science (AAAS)
1776 Massachusetts Avenue, N.W.
Washington, DC 20036
(202) 467-4497 (Voice/TTY)

Handicapping Conditions Served: All handicaps.

The Organization: The Project on the Handicapped in Science was launched in 1975 as the AAAS advocate for disabled professionals and students engaged in science. The Project also acts as an information center for disabled individuals, parents, teachers and employers in areas pertaining to science education and careers. Through surveys, studies, symposia, and workshops, the Project has collected information about science education and employment opportunities for the handicapped in areas requiring science education. Using the information it collects, the Project consults with universities, professional scientific societies, and the Federal government to identify the accessibility and program needs of disabled scientists and students and to suggest strategies to meet those needs.

Information Services: The Project publishes reports, guides, and directories based on its activities, including: *Barrier Free Meetings: A Guide for Professional Associations*, a step-by-step system for achieving accessibility at professional meetings; a *Resource Directory of Handicapped Scientists*, containing names and biographical data of handicapped scientists who will consult with those working to improve science education and career opportunities for handicapped persons; *Science for Handicapped Students in Higher Education*, a summary of findings of Project meetings; *Scientific and Engineering Societies; A Resource for Career Planning*, a listing of counseling, referral, and placement services of scientific professional associations and a source book on career counseling in science; and *A Research Agenda on Science and Technology for the Handicapped*, the findings of a project and workshop researching science and technology for the handicapped.

The Project publishes a quarterly bulletin which reports on the proceedings of workshops on science and technology for the handicapped and the latest developments in technology research.

Registry of Interpreters for the Deaf, Inc. (RID)
814 Thayer Avenue
Silver Spring, MD 20910
(301) 588-2406 (Voice/TTY)

Handicapping Conditions Served: Deafness, hearing impairments and deaf-blindness.

The Organization: The Registry of Interpreters for the Deaf is a membership organization of professional interpreters. Its main purpose is to certify simultaneous (oral and manual) and oral interpreters at various levels of proficiency. RID and its state affiliates actively advocate for the use of interpreters for hearing impaired clients of government and private agencies. Future plans of the Registry include the accreditation of interpreter training programs.

Information Services: RID provides information to interpreters about training programs, professional developments and job opportunities. It publishes a national directory which includes information on certification requirements, bylaws of the organization and professional ethics. Regional directories are regularly updated and contain member listings of interpreters and their certification status as well as teletypewriter agents and vocational rehabilitation specialists.

Brochures are available on various specialties, such as interpreting for teachers, medical interpreting, legal interpreting, law enforcement interpreting, and religious interpreting. Books available from RID include *Sign Language for Interpreters* and a soon to be published book describing interpreter training programs. *Interpreter News*, published bimonthly, contains professional articles, organizational news, training program announcements, and job openings.

Rehabilitation Engineering Society of
**   North America (RESNA)**
1701 South First Avenue
Suite 504
Maywood, IL 60153
(312) 681-2828

Handicapping Conditions Served: All physical handicaps.

The Organization: The Rehabilitation Engineering Society of North America (RESNA) was founded in October 1979 to join together the people participating in the development and delivery of technologies to disabled people with the consumers who benefit from this technology. The Society is concerned with the design, development, evaluation, and production of devices; modification of housing and transportation environments; and creation of an effective delivery system whereby the disabled may receive the benefits of such technology. RESNA's diverse discipline groups will act as task forces to define their own objectives and roles in the delivery process and will interact with each other to assure effective functioning of the delivery system. Such task forces include consumers, health care practitioners, inventors and designers, researchers, manufacturers and distributors, authorizers and providers, and legislators.

Information Services: An organizational brochure and membership information are available from RESNA. The Society plans to publish literature for the lay public and a professional journal.

Part Five

FACILITIES, SCHOOLS, CLINICS

American Printing House for the
Blind (APHB)
1839 Frankfort Avenue
Louisville, KY 40206
(502) 895-2405

Handicapping Conditions Served: Blindness and visual handicaps.

The Organization: Chartered in 1858, the Printing House is the oldest and largest publishing house for the blind in the world. Since 1879 Congressional appropriations have supported publication of textbooks in braille, large print, or recordings for all blind students under college age. In cooperation with the Library of Congress, the Printing House records "Talking Books." APHB also contracts with private agencies or individuals to publish books and periodicals for study or recreational reading by the blind. Other instructional materials produced include more than 250 special educational aids and tools.

A research department conducts basic studies relevant to the education of the blind, and applies this information to the design of new educational materials.

The Printing House has established a central catalog of volunteer produced books which coordinates the services of volunteers who produce a large number of special materials, to make interchange of these materials possible and avoid duplication.

Information Services: Catalogs include braille textbooks, braille recreational reading (fiction, nonfiction, cookbooks, periodicals, music); large type (textbooks, piano tuning, high interest/low vocabulary textbooks, cookbooks); educational aids; talking books, cassette tapes; lists of print books for parents and professionals working with the blind; and brochures describing the Printing House. Information about educational reference materials should be directed to Carl Lappin, Director of the Instructional Materials Reference Center.

Carroll Center for the Blind
770 Centre Street
Newton, MA 02158
(617) 969-6200

Handicapping Conditions Served: Blindness and visual impairments.

The Organization: The Carroll Center for the Blind is a residential and commuter rehabilitation center for visually disabled persons. The Center offers instruction in mobility, handwriting, braille, grooming and other activities of daily living, workshops in woodworking, carpentry and mechanics, and low vision clinic where aids are prescribed and clients are instructed in their usage. Center-trained workers offer instruction in daily living activities to visually handicapped persons in local communities throughout Massachusetts.

Information Services: The Center has developed some free informational materials which it distributes nationally on request. Of interest to workers for the blind, *Aids and Appliances Review* is a quarterly publication which evaluates specific aids and appliances. Other materials include: general information for the newly blinded, elderly blind and blind children; *Sighted Guide,* a manual on ways the sighted person can help the blind; and tips for restaurant employees on serving the blind.

Clovernook Home and School for the Blind
7000 Hamilton Avenue
Cincinnati, OH 45231
(513) 522-3860

Handicapping Conditions Served: Blindness, visual impairments, and deaf-blindness.

The Organization: The Clovernook Home and School for the Blind provides rehabilitation, residential, and work facilities for blind and visually handicapped persons, aged 18 to 55. Work facilities include a sheltered workshop in printing, the **Clovernook Printing House for the Blind**. The Printing House produces braille transcriptions of books, magazines, and other publications for governmental, religious, and nonsectarian organizations, including the Library of Congress.

Information Services: Information about programs of the Clovernook Home is provided free to all inquirers. A list of braille publications produced by the Printing House includes information about where to obtain free braille subscriptions to magazines such as *Better Homes and Gardens, Horizon, Popular Mechanics, Seventeen*, and a variety of religious publications. Copies of magazines which are not distributed through subscription may be obtained from the Printing House. Braille calendars, writing paper, playing cards, and a cookbook are available at nominal costs.

Gallaudet College
Kendall Green
7th and Florida Ave., N.E.
Washington, DC 20002
(202) 651-5000 (voice or TTY)

Handicapping Conditions Served: Hearing impairments, deafness, deaf-blindness.

The Organization: Established by an act of Congress, signed by President Abraham Lincoln in 1864, Gallaudet remains the only accredited liberal arts college for the deaf in the world. The college offers bachelor degree programs in 26 subject areas, master's programs in five, and a Ph.D. in special education administration. Students with normal hearing are admitted as exchange or graduate students, as well as to the two year Associate of Arts program in sign language interpreting. In addition to the College, a Division of Pre-college Programs, a Division of Research, and a Division of Public Services now offer a wide range of services and information in the field of hearing impairments.

Pre-College Programs include the Kendall Demonstration Elementary School for the Deaf (KDES) and the Model Secondary School for the Deaf (MSSD). Both are authorized and funded by Congress to develop and evaluate innovative methods, curricula, and educational technology for the training of deaf children from infancy through secondary school. Both schools are located on Kendall Green and provide opportunity for classroom internships to the Gallaudet college students enrolled in programs of special education of the deaf. MSSD has residential facilities, and accepts students from anywhere in the U.S., while KDES serves day students from the metropolitan Washington, D.C. area. For information on educational research and curricula, contact the MSSD Information Office at Public Relations Office (202) 651-5858 (voice or TTY); or Pre-College Outreach at (202) 651-5048.

Continuing Education: An extensive demonstration program of classes for adults has been developed through the Public Services Division. Curriculum information and assistance in organizing such services is available through the Office of Continuing Education at (202) 651-5597 (voice or TTY).

Sign Language Programs: Instruction in sign language includes training of sign language interpreters. An Associate of Arts degree in interpreting has been developed in cooperation with the National Interpreter Training Consortium and the Registry of Interpreters for the Deaf. Information on curriculum, materials, and standards is available from Dr. Lottie Riekehof at (202) 651-5630 (voice or TTY).

International Center on Deafness: Created in 1974 in response to requests from abroad, the Center offers an individualized program of study to persons from other countries who do not qualify for, or are not interested in pursuing, an academic degree. Application forms and an informational brochure may be requested from the Director (202) 651-5316 (voice or TTY).

The **Research Institute** is a new administrative unit which assists faculty and graduate students develop researchable ideas and explore funding sources. It acts as a clearinghouse for coordination of and collaboration with other research efforts throughout the country. The Institute is also responsible for publication and dissemination of results through a quarterly journal, *Directions*. For further details, contact Doin Hicks at (202) 651-5030.

Gallaudet College Library: Extensive holdings in all subject areas relating to deafness can be obtained through interlibrary loan. Annotated bibliographies may be requested and assistance is available to organizations wishing to develop library services on the subject of deafness. The Gallaudet Media Distribution Service distributes through the library videocassettes, videotapes, and 16 mm. films on sign language instruction, signed educational films, and materials on deafness of interest to the general public as well as parent groups, psychologists, and educators. Catalogs and order forms are available from the library or bookstore. Gallaudet's extensive collection of print and nonprint materials on deafness and communicative disorders is accessible through an in-house computer search system, SIRE-G (Syracuse Information Retrieval Experiment-Gallaudet). Contact the Library for information; there is no cost to users. Requests for bibliographies or other information should be directed to Carolyn Jones, (202) 651-5574.

Office of Demographic Studies: The conduct of national surveys was initiated in 1968 to gather information about hearing impaired children and youth for research by educators, audiologists, psychologists, legislators, and others working in the field of hearing impairments. At present, data are collected on approximately 54,000 students in all types of educational programs throughout the country. Other special projects have included psychological and behavioral studies, and revision of the Stanford Achievement Test for hearing impaired students. Data are available to independent investigators for research purposes, to educational institutions, legislators and other groups devoted to improving education and other services for the hearing impaired. A publication list, bibliographies, and other information are available on request at (202) 651-5300.

National Center for Law and the Deaf: Established in 1975, the Center provides free legal services to the deaf and hearing impaired community. The Center also acts as a clearinghouse of information about court decisions and current litigation associated with deafness, particularly in the area of employment, income maintenance, insurance and tax benefits, and civil rights. Drafts of state and national legislation are prepared at the Center; petitions and briefs for presentation to administrative agencies are also drawn up, as need is indicated. The Center engages in advocacy and initiates class action suits of benefit to hearing impaired citizens. Educational workshops are conducted for groups of deaf and hearing impaired persons to inform them of their legal rights. Assistance is offered to hearing impaired persons in preparing for legal careers. Lay or professional persons, including attorneys, may request information about deaf persons' interests. Brochures explaining services of the center, and a monthly newsletter that reports on legislation affecting the hearing impaired, are available on request. All services are free. Contact the Center for information at (202) 651-5454 (voice or TTY).

Information Services: A quarterly magazine, *Gallaudet Today,* is distributed by the Office of Public Relations. The College Bookstore lists publications and curriculum materials published by the Gallaudet College Press. Each division and program has publications and brochures, describing activities. Inquiries should be directed to the appropriate unit (see telephone numbers under each heading). For general information contact the Office of Alumni and Public Relations (202) 651-5100 (voice or TTY).

Gesell Institute of Human Development
310 Prospect Street
New Haven, CT 06511
(203) 777-3481

Handicapping Conditions Served: Learning and developmental disabilities; visual handicaps; allergies and nutritional problems.

The Organization: Originally the Gesell Institute of Child Development, the Institute changed its name in 1979 and broadened its services to include adults in the medical and visual departments. In the child development clinic, children from two to thirteen are evaluated in a wide range of functions—physical (motor), adaptive, verbal and psycho-personal. Visual therapy is provided and parents of children with developmental difficulties may receive counseling.

The Institute advocates Gesell's philosophy of grouping school children according to behavioral maturation instead of chronological age. When learning disabilities appear to relate to perceptual or nutritional difficulties, appropriate diagnosis and treatment can be given through the Institute's vision and medical departments, or referrals made for treatment at local facilities. A nursery school for preschoolers provides staff members an opportunity for further research in early childhood development and learning. Postgraduate training in diagnosis and treatment of perceptual problems is offered to optometrists on grants from the National Optometric Foundation. Staff members give lectures and workshops at universities throughout the country to explain and help implement Gesell's methods.

Information Services: Brochures describing the services of the Institute, application forms for evaluation, and a publication list of books written by staff members can be requested. On site use of library materials and films is open to interested persons. Professionals, handicapped persons, and their families are welcome to inquire by phone or mail about services, or request referrals to local resources. While most information is free of charge, there is a nominal cost for publications. Fees for direct services vary.

Goodwill Industries of America, Inc.
9200 Wisconsin Avenue, N.W.
Washington, DC 20014
(301) 530-6500

Handicapping Conditions Served: All handicaps.

The Organization: Goodwill Industries began in 1902 when a Boston minister began collecting clothing and household articles for the handicapped in his community to learn to repair; resale of the items financed the operation and gave the workers income as well as job skills. There are now 168 local member organizations and affiliates in 25 countries which offer vocational rehabilitation to over 60,000 handicapped persons annually. Rehabilitation includes testing, job skill training, physical or speech therapy, and counseling of persons with physical or mental handicaps. After job training at Goodwill, many workers are placed in competitive outside employment, but the more severly handicapped are given jobs at home or in sheltered workshops operated by Goodwill. The autonomous member organizations vary in the kind and scope of services offered. Some have developed day nurseries and summer camps; others have housing adapted for the handicapped and aged. Goodwill Industries also works with the federally funded "Projects with Industry" program through which local employers identify specific skills needed, advise on training, and accept placement of trained handicapped workers in such jobs.

Information Services: Manuals, statistical data, audiovisuals and other administrative information, as well as supervision, are available from the national office to assist local organizations or groups interested in establishing new Goodwill centers. Brochures explaining Goodwill services to employers and business contractors may be ordered. A bimonthly newsletter reports activities of local member organizations and legislative developments affecting the handicapped.

Hadley School for the Blind
700 Elm Street
Winnetka, IL 60093
(312) 446-8111

Handicapping Conditions Served: Blindness and deaf-blindness.

The Organization: The Hadley School, which offers correspondence courses free for blind persons, was founded in 1921 by William A. Hadley, a blind high school teacher. The first college level courses were added in the early 1940's. Hadley now has offices in South America, Europe, India, and Africa, offering courses appropriate to the locale and in the native language. Both credit and self improvement courses are offered at no charge to blind or deaf-blind students through braille or cassettes. One-to-one tutoring by correspondence or telephone supplements the lesson materials. Hadley courses are accredited by the North Central Association of Schools and Colleges, and it is possible to earn a high school diploma by correspondence. College courses are arranged in cooperation with the extension services of selected universities and colleges. A two-week intensive training course is offered on site on use of the Optacon, a print reading device.

Information Services: Catalogs in large print or braille list secondary level and self improvement courses ranging from career planning to classical Greek. College level course information can be requested from the Coordinator of the College Program. A Computer Resource Materials Center offers instructional materials and catalogs of braille or tape sources of information in cooperation with Visually Impaired Data Processors International, a group of blind programmers who exchange programs and information to prevent duplication of effort. Library materials on education of the blind and deaf-blind are available to all interested persons for on site research.

Helen Keller National Center for Deaf-Blind
   Youths and Adults
111 Middle Neck Road
Sands Point, NY 11050
(515) 944-8900

Handicapping Conditions Served: Deaf-blindness and accompanying disabilities.

The Organization: Operated by The Industrial Home for the Blind, under an agreement with the Rehabilitation Services Administration of HEW, the Center was authorized by a 1967 Amendment to the Vocational Rehabilitation Act and is funded by annual Congressional appropriations. Extensive evaluative and rehabilitative services are provided to deaf-blind youths and adults, 18 or older. Individualized training in orientation, mobility, communication and life skills, as well as in other areas, is conducted in a residential setting for up to 50 clients at a time, for periods ranging from several months to several years. The training is followed, when appropriate, by specialized job placement and travel orientation. The Center also designs or improves sensory aids to assist the deaf-blind; conducts research in personal adjustment, education and rehabilitation techniques; and offers training to new and prospective rehabilitation specialists who plan to work with the deaf-blind. Eight regional offices provide some financial and consultative assistance to state and local agencies to locate, evaluate, refer or train deaf-blind persons locally. The eight offices, listed in the telephone directories, are found under "Helen Keller National Center" in Sands Point, NY; Philadelphia, PA; Atlanta, GA; Chicago, IL; Dallas, TX; Denver, CO; Seattle, WA; and Glendale, CA.

Information Services: Consultations and referrals may be requested from the national or regional offices. For information on direct services, contact Mr. Louis J. Bettica, Associate Director, at the Helen Keller National Center, or Mr. Dean Wyrick, National Field Services Supervisor, 1111 West Mockingbird Lane, Suite 1540, Dallas, TX 75247. A reference library at the Helen Keller National Center may be used by appointment; copies of some materials are available on loan by special arrangement. Rehabilitation activities of the Center are described in brochures, a newsletter, and a captioned film called "Raising the Curtain."

Pamphlets, fact sheets, bibliographies, indexes and abstracts of articles on deaf-blindness and re-habilitation for professionals and laymen are available. Demographic information and results of the Center's research on personal adjustment, education and rehabilitation may be requested from the research department in New York. Application forms for referral to the Center may be obtained from the local regional office or from the Intake Coordinator, Helen Keller National Center, 111 Middle Neck Road, Sands Point, NY 11050.

Human Resources Center
I. U. Willets Road
Albertson, NY 11507
(516) 747-5400

Handicapping Conditions Served: All physical handicaps and mental retardation.

The Organization: Founded in 1952 by Dr. Henry Viscardi, Jr., a pioneer in the rehabilitation and special education fields, the Human Resources Center is a private, nonprofit organization dedicated to providing educational, vocational, social and recreational opportunities for the severely disabled. The Center's spectrum of programs encompasses job training and placement, academic and vocational education, independent living, research and information dissemination. The Center is composed of three coordinated units: 1) Abilities, Inc., which conducts programs of work evaluation, training, job development and career placement for the disabled, and runs a work demonstration center which employs disabled adults in clerical and industrial operations; 2) Human Resources School, which offers tuition-free education to over 230 severely disabled children; and 3) The Research and Program Development Institute, which conducts research relating to severely disabled persons, initiates and develops demonstration projects in rehabilitation and professional training, and disseminates information and model programs nationally.

In addition, the national Center on Employment of the Handicapped was established in 1977 on the campus of the Human Resources Center with the objective of enhancing employment opportunities for disabled persons through 1) conducting research in such areas as career education, independent living, job placement, and attitudes toward disabled persons; 2) giving seminars and conferences; 3) providing technical assistance; and 4) publishing monographs, textbooks, and multimedia training modules. The nucleus of the national Center on Employment of the Handicapped is the Industry-Labor Council, an outgrowth of the White House Conference on Handicapped Individuals. The Industry-Labor Council unites labor, industry, and rehabilitation, directing efforts toward developing employment opportunities for the handicapped population through serving the needs of the employer community. The Council conducts seminars of interest to employers in the areas of awareness training, affirmative action, and the medical and legal aspects of employment. Technical assistance (consultations, literature distribution, on-site visits, and specialized training) is available to employers. A quarterly newsletter reports on the activities of the Council and its members.

Information Service: The main information dissemination arm of the Human Resources Center is the Research Library, which responds to inquiries on all aspects of the Center's programs and on handicapping conditions and related services. When appropriate, requestors are referred to a staffmember at the Center or to an outside organization. Publications available from the Center include titles on employment, placement, attitudes, driver education, and recreational boating. There is a charge for these publications. Any lay or professional person may request information from the Center. Frequent inquirers include professionals in education and vocational rehabilitation, and members of business and industry.

John Tracy Clinic
806 West Adams Boulevard
Los Angeles, CA 90007
(213) 748-5481

Handicapping Conditions Served: Deafness, hearing impairments, and deaf-blindness.

The Organization: The Clinic is an educational center for deaf and hard-of-hearing preschool children and their parents. One of the Clinic's prime concerns is the training of parents of young hearing impaired children in helping their children to understand language and to speak. Parents may visit or write the Clinic for information, encouragement, and training in coping with a deaf child and in helping the child acquire language, lipreading, and speech skills. Clinic services are available to hearing impaired children and their parents and include: consultation services for the audiological and psychological evaluation of deaf children; parent classes in child development, parent attitudes, and communication skills; psychological counseling for parents; a demonstration nursery school where children and parents are enrolled; summer sessions for parents and children; and a teacher-training course.

Information Services: The Clinic has a library containing books and journals related to deafness, deaf-blindness, and psychological counseling. Educational materials include: *Vocabulary List, Learning to Listen* (an auditory training record); *Play It By Ear* (auditory training games for parents and teachers of young deaf children); *Language Guide* (a detailed description of a 4-year language program for preschool deaf children); *My Child* (helps to explain your child's deafness to others); and special materials for teacher education. In addition, the Clinic publishes a bulletin twice a year.

Correspondence courses for parents of preschool deaf children are offered by the Clinic. They emphasize parent attitudes, communication, motor development, and the teaching of self-care skills. *Getting Your Baby Ready to Talk*, a home study plan for infant language development, is designed for use with the hearing impaired as well as other "high risk" infants whose language development may be inhibited.

All services of the John Tracy Clinic are given free of charge to children and their parents.

Joseph Bulova School of Watchmaking
40-24 62nd Street
Woodside, NY 11377
(212) 424-2929

Handicapping Conditions Served: All physical and emotional handicaps.

The Organization: The Joseph Bulova School of Watchmaking was founded in 1945 to serve returning disabled veterans. Since 1950, the School has accepted disabled civilians, and more recently, nondisabled persons, although 80 percent of its graduates are disabled. The School offers watchmaking, watch repair, and precision technician training on an individualized basis to students. In addition to vocational training and rehabilitation, some job counseling and placement services are offered. Residential students receive health services, counseling, and recreation. Financial aid for tuition and living expenses is available to qualifying students.

Information Services: The Bulova School provides free brochures about its services to any interested person. A film about the school, "To Live On," is available on loan.

**National Institute for
      Rehabilitation Engineering**
97 Decker Road
Butler, NJ 07405
(201) 838-2500
(201) 838-2578 (TTY)

Handicapping Conditions Served: All physical handicaps.

The Organization: The Institute describes itself as a "place of last resort" where medical professionals and engineers combine their expertise to design appliances or technological devices to aid severely handicapped people. Mobility, vision, speech, hearing, and multiple handicaps are among the disabilities for which compensatory aids are developed, but only if other practitioners or clinics have been unable to offer adequate assistance. A multidisciplinary evaluation is made, after which a recommendation is offered which—if accepted by the client—will be implemented by the Institute and, if necessary, the client is trained in the use of the recommended or custom designed appliance. A special low vision driver's training program trains those with specially designed glasses. Internships are available to professionals interested in working with unique and difficult rehabilitation engineering problems. Evaluations and user training are done at the Institute except where special arrangements have been made for alternate locations. Fees are determined on a sliding scale; assistance is offered clients in identifying sources of financial aid when necessary. The Institute has affiliates in England, Sweden, Italy, and Switzerland.

Information Services: Applicants may submit medical and other data for review, without charge. Free information sheets may be requested which describe clinical research services, low vision driver training, hearing aid services, vision aid services and other aids. Membership information and inquiries from professionals should be directed to Don Selwyn, Technical and Training Director. Complex inquiries requiring research and consultation are answered on a fee basis; brief inquiries are answered without charge.

**National Jewish Hospital/
      National Asthma Center (NJH/NAC)**
3800 East Colfax Avenue
Denver, CO 80206
(303) 388-4461

Handicapping Conditions Served: Chronic respiratory and immunologic disorders.

The Organization: In 1978, the National Jewish Hospital and Research Center and the National Asthma Center merged to combine resources. Operating under single management as the NJH/NAC, the institution maintains treatment and research facilities where patients can be referred who need specialized care beyond the means of local facilities. Treatment facilities include medical care and psychological, social, occupational, and recreational therapy for patients with chronic respiratory and immunological diseases. Treatment is available to patients of all ages, beliefs and backgrounds, without regard to their financial circumstances. Family-like living arrangements are provided for pediatric patients. An outpatient program and short-term treatment for children with less severe illnesses are also available. The NJH/NAC facilities blend patient care and research. Areas of NJH/NAC basic research include molecular and cellular biology and specific research in respiratory and immunological diseases. As an affiliate of the University of Colorado Health Sciences Center, NJH/NAC offers a full-time academic program in the allergy field for postgraduate physicians. Short courses are offered in other specialty areas related to respiratory diseases.

Information Services: NJH/NAC publishes four booklets which discuss the causes, diagnosis, and treatment of specific diseases in lay language. They are available free: *Understanding Asthma, Understanding Allergy, Understanding Tuberculosis*, and *Understanding Chronic Bronchitis and Emphysema*. A fifth booklet, *Understanding Immunology*, describes the body's immunological system and possible immunological dysfunctions. A more extensive booklet on asthma, *Your Child and Asthma*, is available for a nominal charge. For additional information, contact Jerry L. Colness, Director of Communications.

National Technical Institute for the Deaf (NTID)
One Lomb Memorial Drive
Rochester, NY 14623
(716) 475-6400

Handicapping Conditions Served: Deafness and severe hearing impairments.

The Organization: The National Technical Institute for the Deaf (NTID) was established by an act of Congress and is funded through the U.S. Department of Health, Education, and Welfare. Since 1968, it has provided a two to three year technical education to deaf and severely hearing impaired students. Staff research in speech therapy, educational methods, and vocational training and placement is reported in professional journals as well as in publications of the Institute. Sign language interpreter training, teaching internships, and workshops for employers, educators, and rehabilitation professionals are offered both on and off campus. The Institute is one of nine colleges of the Rochester Institute of Technology, and "mainstreaming" deaf students in classes elsewhere on campus has been accomplished with significant success.

Information Services: An **Office of Educational Extension** provides curriculum materials; communication packages for speech pathologists; orientation manuals and information on hearing aids for audiologists and consumers; special bibliographies and other data requested by researchers; and the NTID catalog and Institute magazine. An annotated *Mainstreaming Bibliography* in two volumes is a recent product of staff research. There is a nominal charge for most materials.

The **National Center on Employment of the Deaf** at NTID is a newly established office which offers services in employee development, training, continuing education, information services, and career matching. Information and training are available to employers interested in hiring qualified deaf people. Workshops are conducted on site, or employers may attend seminars at NTID. Consulting is also available regarding job analysis, accommodations in the workplace, and access to upward mobility for deaf employees. A career matching system is being developed to match the skills of deaf persons with postsecondary certification to the needs of government, business, and industry on a nationwide basis. Deaf persons and employers will be able to make use of this system. Training and consulting are also provided for placement professionals working with deaf persons concerning successful placement strategies for qualified deaf persons.

Perkins School for the Blind
175 N. Beacon Street
Watertown, MA 02172
(617) 924-3434

Handicapping Conditions Served: Blindness, deaf-blindness, and multi-handicapped blind.

The Organization: The Perkins School was chartered in 1829 to educate blind and deaf-blind children. It is a private residential school, serving blind students, and clients age 0-adult and is accredited to award a high school diploma. Additional services include a rehabilitation program in which older persons or Perkins School graduates learn daily living and employment skills; a nonresidential preschool; a special program for learning disabled blind children; and the deaf-blind program. A teacher training program is offered in cooperation with Boston College. The Howe Press, a division of Perkins, manufactures the Perkins Brailler as well as other appliances and materials for blind students. A historical museum on campus is open to the public. While Perkins is a private school, tuition is usually paid by the state or local agency which refers the student.

Information Services: The Howe Memorial Press of the Perkins School has lists of curriculum materials and of publications for educators and parents including a *Bibliography of the Deaf-Blind, Speech Beginnings for the Deaf-Blind Child,* and the *Perkins Sign Language Directory*. Price lists for appliances (including the Braille typewriter), and for publications are available on request. Public education films, brochures, and books are available from the public relations office; there is a nominal charge for some materials. A research library is open for on site use.

Rubella Project
Developmental Disabilities Center
St. Luke's Roosevelt Hospital Center
428 West 59th Street
New York, NY 10019
(212) 554-6565

Handicapping Conditions Served: Rubella.

The Organization: The Rubella Project was established for research, training and service in prevention and management of rubella and congenital rubella, and for research in rubella vaccines. The Project provides medical and allied services to children with congenital rubella in the New York metropolitan area and is a national referral center for unusual complications associated with rubella and rubella vaccines.

Information Services: The Rubella Project responds to telephone and mail inquiries related to the disease and current management techniques. It makes referrals to diagnostic centers located in the northeastern U.S. A bibliography of scientific articles on rubella is available from the Project.

Sister Kenny Institute
Division of Abbott-Northwestern Hospital
Chicago Avenue at 27th Street
Minneapolis, MN 55407
(612) 874-4149

Handicapping Conditions Served: Musculoskeletal and neurological disorders.

The Organization: The Institute was established in 1941 by Sister Kenny, an Australian nurse who revolutionized the treatment for polio. Her method has been adapted and treatment expanded to include comprehensive rehabilitation for victims of spinal cord injury, stroke, or other disorders affecting movement. Since 1975 the Institute has been a division of Abbott-Northwestern Hospital, where it takes over the care of patients coming out of the acute care facility and offers a continuum of rehabilitative services. Departments include occupational, recreational, and physical therapy; speech pathology and audiology; a day care center; a residential treatment center for chronic pain, and neuroaugmentive surgery, a new technique for its relief; vocational rehabilitation, job placement, psychological, and social services. A department of research and education offers both graduate and continuing education courses for health professionals in long term care, nursing, and rehabilitation. These courses can be given at other locations by arrangement.

Information Services: A wide variety of health care materials are prepared and published by the Institute for health professionals, patients, and their families. The catalog lists publications and audiovisuals on home care, clothing and travel, speech therapy, care of ostomies, diabetes, physical therapy, and other aspects of rehabilitation. Information about publications and courses may be obtained from Dr. Joseph Kent Canine.

**Trace Research and Development Center
for the Severely Communicatively
Handicapped**
314 Waisman Center
1500 Highland Avenue
Madison, WI 53706
(608) 262-6966

Handicapping Conditions Served: Severe speech impairments.

The Organization: In cooperation with the Communication Aids and Systems Clinic of the University of Wisconsin, the Center studies available techniques and aids, or develops appropriate ones, to augment whatever vocal skills may be available to a clinic patient. The Center collects, documents, and disseminates information on these and other communication aids and techniques to interested professionals and others in the U.S. and abroad. To eliminate duplication of effort and promote compatible material and aids, the Center works to inventory and coordinate research efforts among others in this rapidly growing field. Efforts are also made to facilitate commercial production of special materials and aids, to increase availability.

Information Services: The Center publishes the *Non-Vocal Communication Resource Book* with semiannual updates available on a subscription basis. A reprint service includes information on recent developments in communication technology and techniques. With the Artificial Language Laboratory at Michigan State University, the Center publishes a quarterly newsletter, *Communication Outlook*. On site use of the Center's library is available to any interested researchers. There is a nominal charge for most publications, but much information is available at no cost.

Part Six

SERVICE ORGANIZATIONS

All Federal Agencies are asterisked for easy identification.

Page

**Adventures in Movement for
   Handicapped Kids (AIM)**
945 Danbury Road
Dayton, OH 45420
(513) 294-4611

Handicapping Conditions Served: All handicaps.

The Organization: Adventures in Movement for Handicapped Kids (AIM) was founded in 1958 to promote the teaching of movement using the AIM method, a series of rhythmical exercises involving gross and fine motor movements. The purpose of the method is to improve muscle control and coordination, and thereby enhance self-image. The program can be adapted for instruction to all handicapped persons and all age groups. The organization's major activity is the training of classroom teachers and volunteers in the AIM method. Workshops are planned to meet the particular needs of sponsoring groups.

Information Services: Brochures describe the AIM method and the organization's workshops. A handbook, *Adventures in Movement for the Handicapped,* illustrates the exercises used in AIM classes. "Maybe Tomorrow," a film of the AIM method in actual classroom use, is available for rent or purchase. The organization will provide a list of school systems with AIM programs upon request. For further information, contact Carolyn Kirkwood, Educational Director.

Aid to Adoption of Special Kids (AASK)
3530 Grand Avenue
Suite 202
Oakland, CA 94610
(415) 451-1748

Handicapping Conditions Served: All handicaps.

The Organization: Aid to Adoption of Special Kids (AASK) helps to place older children, sibling groups, minority children, and emotionally, mentally, and physically handicapped children in permanent homes. AASK is licensed as an adoption agency in the States of California and Nevada. It serves the national adoption scene by acting as an intermediary between adoption agencies and parents seeking to adopt "special kids."

Information Services: AASK maintains files of available children, referred by caseworkers or adoption agencies throughout the U.S., and a registry of families seeking to adopt difficult to place children. When AASK can match a request of adoptive parents with a specific child listed in its files, the parents are referred to the appropriate adoption agency. Individual requests for information on the availability and needs of adoptable handicapped children, financial resources available to adoptive families, and proper adoption procedures are answered by phone or letter.

American Camping Association
Bradford Woods
Martinsville, IN 46151
(317) 342-8456

Handicapping Conditions Served: All handicaps.

The Organization: The Association inspects and accredits camps throughout the country according to standards of hygiene, safety, and program. An annual guide for parents lists camps which mainstream physically or mentally retarded children, and others which serve epileptics, diabetics, asthmatics, learning disabled, deaf, blind, and physically, emotionally, or mentally handicapped children, youths, and adults. The primary focus of the Association, however, is not on services to the handicapped.

Information Services: *Camping Magazine* is the official journal of the Association. The annual *Parents Guide to Accredited Camps* is published for four areas: northeast, south, midwest and west. Contact Lois Lehr at the Association office for additional information.

American National Red Cross
17th and D Streets, N.W.
Washington, DC 20006
(202) 737-8300

Handicapping Conditions Served: All handicaps.

The Organization: The American National Red Cross was established in 1881 by Clara Barton. Some of its areas of service are disaster relief, blood programs, services to military personnel and their families, safety, and nursing and health programs. The handicapped are given priority transportation., shelter, food, clothing, and medical assistance in case of disaster. Through 3100 local chapters, and depending on the needs of the community, volunteers offer transportation services, hot meal programs, and assistance at community rehabilitation and recreation centers for the handicapped. In addition to programs initiated at the local level, the national office has designed programs for the handicapped which are implemented by the chapters.

A program of **Adapted Aquatics** is offered to all handicapped persons, in cooperation with community agencies. The Red Cross trains swimming instructors to teach the handicapped. Many aquatic and first aid materials are available in braille and large print.

First Things First, an 8-week program given in schools, teaches basic first aid skills to the educable mentally retarded and those with learning disabilities. Youth Services has also designed a **Deaf Awareness Program** to train volunteers and school personnel in involving deaf and hearing people in voluntary services to the community.

A **Multiple Sclerosis Home Care Course** is offered to nurses and volunteers through local Red Cross and National Multiple Sclerosis Society chapters.

Information Services: Books, manuals, and audiovisuals on adapted aquatics, and training kits and films from each of the Youth Services programs (First Things First and the Deaf Awareness Program) are available. A booklet, *Opportunities for Youth in the American Red Cross*, which contains volunteer activities for the handicapped, and a complete publications catalog are available. Publications may be requested from local chapters—some chapters also publish their own materials.

A Chapter Program Exchange in the Community Volunteer Services office at national headqarters serves as a clearinghouse for information about direct services provided by each chapter. The Office of Safety Services has information about the chapters that have braille or cassette copies of *Standard First Aid and Personal Safety*.

Amputee Shoe and Glove Exchange
Dr. and Mrs. R. E. Wainerdi
1635 Warwickshire Drive
Houston, TX 77077

Handicapping Conditions Served: Amputation.

The Organization: The Amputee Shoe and Glove Exchange provides a free service to facilitate the exchange of unneeded shoes and gloves among amputees.

Information Services: The Exchange maintains a list of amputees with information on their age, size, style preferences, and size needed. This information is then sent to an amputee with similar tastes and the opposite side amputated. All mailings of shoes or gloves are between the amputees themselves.

Association of Radio Reading Services (ARRS)
1745 University Avenue
St. Paul, MN 55104
(612) 296-6034

Handicapping Conditions Served: Visual and physical handicaps.

The Organization: The Association of Radio Reading Services was established in 1977 to promote the growth of such services throughout the country, and to provide for the development and sharing of advanced technology and for a unified effort in pursuit of legislation supportive of Radio Reading Services.

Radio Reading Services are independently operated broadcasts of news and information for visually and physically handicapped persons who cannot read printed materials for themselves. Broadcasts are presented by trained volunteers and include readings of newspapers, magazines and books. Now on the air in about 70 communities throughout the U.S., these services operate on a closed channel basis (an FM station simultaneously broadcasts the service along with its regular programming to designated listeners who are provided special receivers) or an open channel basis (local stations interrupt their regular programming for the service and special receiver equipment is not required).

Information Services: ARRS publishes informational brochures on Radio Reading Services and how to establish them. Memos on issues affecting the broadcasts of special programs, such as regulations of the Federal Communications commission or the Office of Telecommunications, are periodically distributed to member services. Information is available about possible funding sources and broadcast and receiver equipment. ARRS will provide on-site consultation or referrals to other consultants.

B'nai B'rith Career and Counseling
Services (BBCCS)
1640 Rhode Island Avenue, N.W.
Washington, DC 20036
(202) 393-5284

Handicapping Conditions Served: All handicaps.

The Organization: The B'nai B'rith Career and Counseling Service (BBCCS) offers counseling to youths facing career choices and to adults who face vocational adjustment problems, second-career choices, or retirement. BBCCS has 20 facilities across the country which offer individual and group counseling services. Individual counseling is offered mainly to Jewish youth and adults, but group sessions are open to the community. Most group programs are relevant to all persons, including the handicapped, who are seeking careers, jobs, or schools.

Information Services: A catalog of publications includes literature and directories for counselors, parents, and students. Opportunities in various professional fields are reviewed in an occupational brief series. Of particular interest to the handicapped are these special publications: *Student Aids in the Space Age: Educational Resources for the Handicapped; Careers for the Homebound: Home Study Educational Opportunities; Small Business as a Rehabilitative Technique for the Aging;* and *Space Age Challenges and New Career Horizons for the Deaf.* The *1978-79 College Guide for Jewish Youth* lists special facilities for handicapped college students with visual, hearing, or mobility impairments.

Boy Scouts of America
Scouting for the Handicapped Service
P.O. Box 61030
Dallas-Ft. Worth Airport, TX 75261
(214) 659-2108

Handicapping Conditions Served: All handicaps.

The Organization: Scouting for the Handicapped is designed to include young handicapped people in regular units or in groups at schools and homes for handicapped youth, when inclusion in ongoing scouting activities is not possible. National voluntary organizations with expertise in specific handicapping conditions assist Scouting for the Handicapped in devising special programs and materials.

Information Services: Audiovisual and print publications for scout leaders contain specific activities for handicapped scouts and ways to involve the handicapped in regular scouting activities. Scouting manuals are available on the mentally retarded, the physically handicapped, the deaf, and the visually handicapped. For visually impaired scouts, a list of braille scouting books and their suppliers is available from the Service. A general bibliography of reading for mentally retarded boys is also available. All information is provided free.

Child Welfare League of America (CWLA)
67 Irving Place
New York, NY 10003
(212) 254-7410

Handicapping Conditions Served: All handicaps.

The Organization: The Child Welfare League of America (CWLA) is a federation of about 400 public and private social service agencies in Canada and the U.S. which provide a variety of child welfare services to children and their families. The agencies' services include, but are not limited to, foster care, counseling, day care, adoption, and services for unmarried parents. The League offers consultation to agencies on day-to-day and long range problems in policy, program, and practice. It establishes standards, provides consultation, conducts research, holds regional workshops and training conferences for professionals, offers a personnel referral service, and acts as an advocate for child welfare.

Among the League's several specialized programs is the **North American Center on Adoption (NACA)**, which encourages—through advocacy, professional training, and public information—adoption of difficult to place children (older, handicapped, or minority children). The Adoption Resource Exchange of North America (ARENA) is the outreach arm of NACA.

Under a separate grant from HEW, CWLA is conducting a developmental disabilities project which focuses on the adoption of the severely handicapped. Data on agencies with success in placing children with developmental disabilities will be collected and published in monograph form. CWLA plans to train agency staff in placing the developmentally disabled.

Through grants from HEW, the League has developed three curricula for **foster parent education**: Introduction to Foster Parenting; Foster Parenting a Retarded Child; and Foster Parenting an Adolescent. Brochures detailing the materials, and consultation on the use of the materials are available upon request.

Information Services: The League's Library/Information Service acts as a clearinghouse for information about child welfare services and related subjects. It has a national videotaped lending library for agencies, organizations, and individuals.

The ARENA office refers parents to local adoption agencies and advises parents on problems they may have in the adoption process.

A publication catalog includes titles of more than 120 books on foster parenting and administration of foster care agencies. Final reports on League studies are also available. CWLA publishes a professional journal, *Child Welfare*, as well as newsletters covering administrative, legislative, and parenting topics. Among those periodicals, *ARENA News* is particularly relevant to the field of the handicapped since it provides pictures and descriptive profiles from the ARENA list of waiting children as well as articles related to foster care of hard to place children.

For additional information, contact William G. Moore, Director, Public Information.

Clothing Research and Development Foundation (CRDF)
P.O. Box 347
Milford, NJ 08848

Handicapping Conditions Served: All physical handicaps.

The Organization: The Clothing Research and Development Foundation was founded to help alleviate the clothing problems of the physically handicapped for whom daily dressing is a major effort. Currently, CRDF educates and consults with designers and manufacturers on clothing designs which will permit handicapped persons to dress themselves without aid or with minimal aid.

Information Services: Information about types of clothing for the disabled and sources where they may be obtained is available from CRDF. For professionals, a *Bibliography on Clothing for the Disabled*, produced by the Institute of Rehabilitation Medicine of the New York University Medical Center, is also available from the Foundation.

Eye-Bank Association of America (EBAA)
3195 Maplewood Avenue
Winston-Salem, NC 27103
(919) 768-0719

Handicapping conditions Served: Blindness and visual impairments.

The Organization: The main purpose of eye-banks is to secure eye tissue and to preserve it until it is needed for eye transplants. The Eye-Bank Association of America (EBAA) was founded in 1961 by the **American Academy of Opthalmology and Otolaryngology (AAOO)** for the purpose of promoting and standardizing eye-banks. EBAA has 66 associated eye-bank members, which meet the criteria set by the Association's medical advisory committee. This committee also certifies technicians working in eye-banks.

Information Services: The Association distributes promotional materials to its eye-bank members intended to inform the public of the needs of eye-banks. EBAA answers inquiries from the public on how to donate eyes for corneal surgery. Films are available on a rental basis on removal of eyes for preservation and the technical operation of eye-banks. EBAA publishes abstracts of papers delivered at the annual meetings of EBAA and the AAOO.

Girl Scouts of the U.S.A.
830 Third Avenue
New York, NY 10022
(212) 940-7500

Handicapping Conditions Served: All handicaps.

The Organization: Activities of the Girl Scouts are open to all girls, aged 6 to 17, able-bodied and disabled. Some of the 350 Girl Scout Councils actively recruit girls with disabilities into regular scouting activities. Where mainstreaming into regular troops is not possible, some Councils have established troops at residential homes and schools for the handicapped. The national office estimates that there are more than 20,000 girls with special needs who participate in Girl Scout troops across the country.

Information Services: The Girl Scouts organization publishes various literature including the following specific materials relating to girls with disabilities: *Girl Scout Program: Accessible to All Girls*; and *Serving Girls with Special Needs,* a series of six articles reprinted from *Girl Scout Leader Magazine.*

International Handicappers' Net
PO Box B
San Gabriel, CA 91778
(213) 282-0014

Handicapping Conditions Served: All handicaps.

The Organization: Any handicapped person (including the deaf, blind and mute, who operate radios using the Continental Code) who is a qualified amateur radio operator is eligible for membership in the International Handicappers' Net. The international membership of 2400 communicates via radio at the appointed frequency (14287 KHz upper sideband) at 1600 Greenwich Time (1500 during daylight savings time), Monday through Friday. While members use the Net for communicating with other members, they also handle public service messages and are trained to handle emergency communication in the event of disasters.

Information Services: Information about the organization is provided to any inquirer upon request. New members are referred to members in their locales for assistance and information about the operation. There is no fee for membership.

Just One Break, Inc. (J.O.B.)
373 Park Avenue South
New York, New York 10016
(212) 725-2500

Handicapping Conditions Served: All physical handicaps.

The Organization: J.O.B. was founded in 1949, to assist disabled veterans of World War II reenter the job market. It now serves any persons with a physical disability who is seeking full-time competitive employment. Interviews, group job seeking skills sessions, resume preparation, and other individualized placement services are offered at no charge to the applicant or employer. The organization also carries out research studies in the placement of handicapped workers, and conducts demonstration projects relating to employment of the disabled. While actual placement services are usually limited to the metropolitan New York area, information on employment of handicapped persons is disseminated nationwide—to employers, rehabilitation centers, medical facilities, educational institutions, veterans' hospitals, training centers, and charitable groups. Public awareness activities include the publication of articles and speeches to interested groups. A special program of placement services for blind and visually impaired workers is underway.

Information Services: J.O.B. publishes a quarterly description of the qualifications of available job applicants for 3,000 interested New York area employers. Brochures describing the organization's services, and an annual report summarizing the year's activities are available on request. A manual describing the operations of J.O.B. is available to agencies interested in establishing a similar organization elsewhere in the country. J.O.B. is preparing a textbook on job placement of the disabled to be used in university rehabilitation counseling programs.

Legal Services Corporation
733 15th Street, N.W.
Washington, DC 20005
(202) 272-4000

Handicapping Conditions Served: All handicaps.

The Organization: The Legal Services Corporation was set up by Congress to support local legal services for the poor. The Research Institute on Legal Assistance, part of the Corporation, conducts research activities through a permanent staff and a fellowship program. Research topics being explored include: Health, including Medicaid and Medicare; nursing homes; hospital services for the poor; after-care; services for the mentally retarded; Social Security; and family law and child abuse. The Institute also conducts seminars and meetings on topics that affect the law and on services needed by the poor.

Information Services: Handicapped individuals confronting legal problems who meet financial eligibility guidelines can get services at no cost from the approximately 335 Legal Services programs operating in neighborhood offices throughout the nation. The Institute sponsors a fellowship program every year whereby individuals (for the most part in the law professions) work on special legal research problems. Examples of the types of studies conducted and published by the Institute are: *The New Clients: Legal Services for Mentally Retarded Persons,* a monograph on legal issues affecting mentally retarded persons and the kind of actions needed to serve this population; and a study on special access difficulties and special legal problems of the elderly and handicapped, to be published in early 1980.

Louis Braille Foundation
  for Blind Musicians (LBF)
215 Park Avenue South
New York, NY 10003
(212) 982-7290

Handicapping Conditions Served: Blindness.

The Organization: The Louis Braille Foundation for Blind Musicians (LBF) provides vocational training assistance, vocational counseling, and job placement to enable talented blind musicians to compete on an equal footing with their sighted colleagues. LBF auditions and counsels artists, arranges for appropriate training, provides scholarships to supplement other resources, provides musical instruments and special equipment, and copyrights original musical works for blind composers. The LFB Artists Bureau obtains paid engagements, sponsors concerts to present talented blind artists, and provides publicity services to professionals.

Information Services: The Foundation provides hand produced braille transcriptions of music. A Foundation brochure is also available upon request.

National Braille Association (NBA)
654-A Godwin Avenue
Midland, NJ 07432
(201) 447-1484

Handicapping Conditions Served: Blindness and visual impairments.

The Organization: The National Braille Association (NBA) is an organization of professional and volunteer workers for the blind which publishes and distributes braille textbooks for college and graduate students and educational materials for braille transcribers. The Braille Book Bank provides thermoform duplicates of textbooks, music manuscripts, and statistical tables to students at regular textbook costs. Its collection contains more than 1500 titles. Individual requests for braille transcription of materials such as recipes, and instructions for using tools or for daily living activities are met, as volunteers are available to transcribe them. The Association conducts regular workshops in such specialty areas as braille music, teaching braille transcribing, math-science transcribing, and tactile illustrating.

Information Services: The Braille Book Bank catalogs are available free in print or braille form. NBA provides information to transcribers about current format, transcription codes and practices recognized by the Library of Congress. Professional publications include manuals on braille transcription of mathematics, foreign languages, computer notations, and music. Manuals on large type and tape recording transcribing are also available. For further information, contact Mrs. Doris Ensle, National Office Secretary.

National Captioning Institute, Inc. (NCI)
5203 Leesburg Pike, Suite 1500
Falls Church, VA 22041
(703) 998-2400 (Voice)
(703) 820-2230 (TTY)

Handicapping Conditions Served: Deafness and hearing impairments

The Organization: The National Captioning Institute (NCI) is a nonprofit organization whose function is to caption television programs for broadcast on the Public Broadcasting Service (PBS) and the commercial networks. PBS has played a major role in developing the caption system. NCI was established with funding from HEW's Bureau of Educaton for the Handicapped. The Institute's primary goal is to make captioned television available to every deaf and hearing-impaired person who wants it.

Closed captioning is a system that converts the TV program sound track into words or captions that are shown on the viewer's television screen. The captions are coded and transmitted by the broadcaster on a portion of the television frame that does not ordinarily carry picture information. Unlike open captions which are seen by all viewers, closed captions are seen only on television sets equipped with a special device. The equipment needed to receive closed captions is manufactured and marketed by Sears, Roebuck & Co. By the end of 1980, a substantial number of captioned programs—predominantly prime time—will be broadcast each week. An increase in the number of captioned programs broadcast by the networks and local TV stations will depend largely on the demand by television viewers for the special equipment.

Information Services: The Institute provides information on the history of the Captioning Project and the activities of NCI. Catalogs of educational and commercial captioned films are available from the Captioned Films Distribution Center (see Conference of Executives of American Schools for the Deaf).

National 4-H Council
7100 Connecticut Avenue
Washington, DC 20015
(301) 656-9000

Handicapping Conditions Served: All handicaps.

The Organization: The National 4-H Council is a private organization devoted to the advancement of 4-H work. It was established to contribute to the development of youth as responsible and productive citizens. While the 4-H does not have a national program for the handicapped, many special programs are undertaken by local 4-H groups to involve handicapped youth in activities such as gardening, animal projects, mechanics, sewing, horseback riding, and many more. Instruction in food and nutrition and automobile and bicycle safety is offered to the handicapped by 4-H leaders in some communities. Some programs are conducted in special institutions.

Information Services: Since 4-H projects and publications are developed at the state and local levels, informational materials from the national office are limited. Handicapped youth interested in special services are referred to their local 4-H groups for information. Locally developed publications available from the national office include: *Let's Take a Look at 4-H and Handicapped Youth, Recreation and Handicapped Youth,* and *You Can Hear Me If You Try.* These publications are mainly for group leaders but are available to anyone and are free.

National Industries for the Blind (NIB)
320 Fulton Avenue
Hempstead, NY 11550
(516) 485-0230

Handicapping Conditions Served: Blindness.

The Organization: National Industries for the Blind (NIB) was established in 1938 to act as the designated liaison between workshops for the blind and Federal Government procurement representatives (see separate entry for Committee for Purchase from the Blind and Other Severely Handicapped). Approximately 100 workshops, employing more than 5,000 blind and multihandicapped blind persons, are associated with NIB, and their activities involve producing goods and services for government and private industry. NIB's main functions are to allocate Government Purchase Orders among qualified workshops and to provide training and consultation to workshop boards and personnel in the areas of workshop management, mechanical and industrial engineering, quality assurance, product research and development, vocational rehabilitation services and subcontract procurement. NIB works with new workshops—helping them to meet the special requirements of both NIB and the Committee—and with representatives in industry to create employment opportunities for blind persons. There are no fees or dues for association with NIB.

Information Services: Information available through NIB relates to the standards and requirements for association with NIB, as well as assistance in establishing new workshops for blind and multihandicapped blind persons. General information about NIB and a list of associated workshops are available to any individual.

National Industries for the Severely Handicapped (NISH)
4350 East-West Highway
Suite 1120
Washington, DC 20014
(301) 654-0115

Handicapping Conditions Served: All handicaps, when severe.

The Organization: National Industries for the Severely Handicapped (NISH) was organized in 1974 by a coalition of private agencies long connected with handicapped individuals and workshops. These agencies established NISH to act as the designated liaison between workshops and Federal Government procurement representatives (see separate entry for Committee for Purchase from the Blind and Other Severely Handicapped). NISH has three major functions: 1) to identify commodities and services which are feasible for production in sheltered workshops employing the severely handicapped; 2) to assist workshops in meeting legal requirements; and 3) to evaluate and assist individual sheltered workshops to produce and manage Federal contracts. More than 800 workshops are associated with NISH; more than 100 are producing items or providing services for the Federal Government.

Information Services: An information packet outlines the preliminary steps involved in setting up a workshop and provides information about the Javits-Wagner-O'Day Act and the kind of assistance NISH offers. A *Workshop Manual* details NISH performance standards. Other publications include: *Job Placement Study*, a report on factors affecting the placement of employees from sheltered workshops into competitive industry; and *Basic Procedures for Selling Commodities and Services to the Federal Government, A Guide for Sheltered Workshops*.

New Eyes for the Needy
549 Millburn Avenue
Short Hills, NJ 07078
(201) 376-4903

Handicapping Conditions Served: Visual impairments.

The Organization: New Eyes for the Needy provides funds for new prescription glasses, artificial eyes, and lenticular contact lenses (for cataract patients) to medically indigent persons who are not eligible for other sources of financial assistance. New Eyes solicits metal frames in any condition, unbroken plastic frames with single vision lenses, sunglasses, brown artificial eyes, cataract lenses, soft eyeglass cases, and any precious metal scrap such as old jewelry or silverware. The organization ships reusable glasses to medical missions and welfare agencies abroad for redistribution. Metal framed glasses and metal scrap are sent to be refined, and the proceeds furnish the funds to provide glasses for the needy in the U.S.

Information Services: New Eyes has organizational brochures describing its history, function, how a community group can organize a collection drive, and how donors should package and send materials to New Eyes. Information about qualifying for financial assistance from New Eyes is given to lay and medical inquirers.

Organization for Use of the Telephone,
Inc. (OUT)
Post Office Box 175
Owings Mills, MD 21117
(301) 655-1827

Handicapping Conditions Served: Hearing impaired.

The Organization: The Organization for Use of the Telephone (OUT) was founded in 1973 as a consumer advocacy group for the hearing impaired. Its main concern, as its name implies, is to make the telephone an accessible instrument of communication to those who are "phone deaf." To this end, OUT has held a major role in persuading telephone companies to convert both public and home phones to make them electronically compatible with telephone pick-ups in hearing aids. At this writing, there are about 130 million hearing aid compatible phones in the U.S.; 35 to 40 million are incompatible.

OUT is also an active advocate for the installation of Induction Loop Amplification (ILA) systems in places of public gatherings. Induction loops, when used with hearing aid telephone pick-ups, provide added amplification and clarity to the hearing impaired, making hearing and understanding possible without the need for lipreading.

Information Services: OUT provides inquirers with organizational materials, information on the use of hearing aids with telephones, and copies of relevant news articles, congressional bills and testimony. The *OUT-Line*, published quarterly, informs the membership and other interested persons of national and local efforts to improve communication technology for the hearing impaired. Individual mail and phone inquiries relating to problems with telephone usage are answered by OUT. OUT intervenes with telephone companies to acquire compatible phones for hearing aid users. All information is provided free.

People to People Committee
for the Handicapped
1522 K Street, N.W.
Room 1130
Washington, DC 20005
(202) 638-2487

Handicapping Conditions Served: All handicaps.

The Organization: The People to People Committee for the Handicapped exchanges information about technical developments and programs for the handicapped between organizations in the U.S. and similar groups in other countries. The Committee provides technical assistance to developing countries in setting up rehabilitation facilities for the handicapped, and donates equipment to handicapped persons throughout the world.

Information Services: The Committee publishes the *Directory of Organizations Interested in the Handicapped* containing lists and abstracts of national organizations involved in services to the handicapped. Special project activities of the Committee are reported in a series entitled *Developments in Services for Handicapped People.* A quarterly newsletter reports on current developments in programs for the handicapped and on relevant Federal legislation. All information is provided free.

Recording for the Blind (RFB)
215 East 58th Street
New York, NY 10022
(212) 751-0860

Handicapping Conditions Served: Blindness and visual impairments; physical and perceptual handicaps that in any way prevent the person from reading normal printed material.

The Organization: Recording for the Blind (RFB) supplies taped educational books in open reel and cassette form, free on loan to handicapped students whose objective is to earn diplomas and academic degrees. RFB also serves adults who require specialized taped educational materials to maintain business and professional roles. RFB accepts special requests to tape textbooks which are not already contained in its Master Tape Library. Those titles are then added to the library's 50,000 titles at the average rate of 350 each month.

Information Services: A 1979 RFB catalog of master tapes is available at minimal charge in print form. Each year a supplement to the catalog is printed.

Ruth Rubin Feldman National
Odd Shoe Exchange
3100 Neilson Way—220
Santa Monica, CA 90405
(213) 392-4416

Handicapping Conditions Served; Polio, amputation, and other foot disorders.

The Organization: The Exchange serves persons who need only one shoe or whose shoe requirements are different for each foot. It acts as a clearinghouse to bring together those persons with complementary shoe needs who have serviceable shoes to exchange.

Information Services: The exchange does not deal with shoes, but provides the names of persons of similar ages and tastes in shoe styles. Individuals make their own arrangements for the exchange of shoes and for the purchase of future pairs. An annual membership fee of $5.00 is required to register with the Exchange.

Shriners Hospitals for Crippled Children
2900 Rocky Point Drive
Tampa, FL 33623
(813) 885-2575

Handicapping Conditions Served: Children's orthopedic or burn disabilities.

The Organization: The Shriners' first children's orthopedic hospital opened in 1922, as the official philanthropy of the fraternal order. There are now 18 Orthopedic Hospitals and three Burn Institutes serving children up to age 18 in the U.S., Mexico, and Canada. Diagnosis and treatment are offered solely on the basis of medical and financial need, at no charge to the patient's family. The Burn Institutes accept children who need immediate care or those needing plastic surgery and rehabilitation ("healed" burns). Research on the causes of crippling and scarring and on methods of treatment is conducted at each Shrine Hospital. Members' assessments, charitable bequests, and a variety of fund raising activities support this network of patient care and research facilities.

Information Services: Application forms for hospital admission, information brochures on the hospitals and burn institutes, donation and bequest forms are available from local Shrine Temples or from the International Headquarters. Eligibility for treatment is determined on the basis of applications which are completed by parents or guardians, the referring physician, and a local Shrine sponsor. For emergency admission to burn institutes or hospitals, call Shriners Hospitals for Crippled Children in Tampa, FL, (813) 885-2575.

Telecommunications for the Deaf, Inc. (TDI)
814 Thayer Avenue
Silver Spring, MD 20910
(301) 588-4605 (Voice)
(301) 589-3006 (TTY)

Handicapping Conditions Served: Deafness, hearing impairments, deaf-blindness, and speech impairments.

The Organization: Telecommunications for the Deaf, Inc. (TDI) acquires teletypewriters (TTYs) which are no longer in use from donor sources such as telephone companies and Western Union. TDI's approved agents across the country adapt and install the equipment for the deaf to use in their homes as telephone communication. TDI supports legislation affecting TTY users, especially tax legislation that will lower rates for TTY calls. TDI is also trying to secure the installation TTYs in public places.

Information Services: TDI publishes the *International Telephone Directory of the Deaf* which includes the TTY numbers of agencies and organizations that serve the deaf and individuals who are members of TDI. Nominal dues entitle members to a listing in the Directory and to an organizational newsletter. TDI refers individuals to approved local agents who sell and install TTYs.

Volunteer Services for the Blind (VSB)
919 Walnut Street
Philadelphia, PA 19107
(215) 627-0600

Handicapping Conditions Served: Blindness, visual impairments, and deaf-blindness.

The Organization: Volunteer Services for the Blind (VSB) provides braille, large type, and recordings of a variety of reading material to blind and partially sighted persons. VSB also transcribes materials for government agencies, including the Library of Congress. Each Fall, VSB offers a braille transcriber training program free for those who wish to do volunteer transcribing. Persons who successfully complete the course are certified by the Library of Congress, National Library Service for the Blind and Physically Handicapped. VSB trains handicapped persons to use the Optacon (a tactile scanning device that "reads" print), and makes the device available at cost.

Information Services: More than 200 volunteers across the country transcribe textbooks, professional materials, music, and recreational materials. VSB regularly records certain magazines and journals, and will fill individual requests for periodicals not available from other sources. Braille-transcribed materials are provided free, except for those transcribed by a computer (nominal charge). A list of recorded periodicals is available; periodicals must be subscribed to and are on a loan basis.

APPENDICES

RELIGIOUS ORGANIZATIONS SERVING THE HANDICAPPED

American Bible Society (ABS)
1865 Broadway
New York, NY 10023
(212) 581-7400

The American Bible Society (ABS) translates, produces, and distributes the nondenominational Bible, in whole or in part, for handicapped persons who cannot read or understand regular editions of the Bible. Materials include: embossed Scriptures, talking Bible records, recordings of the New Testament and Psalms, and large print materials for the blind and visually impaired; Bible stories illustrated in American Sign Language for deaf youths; and Scriptures in simplified language for mentally retarded individuals.

Braille Circulating Library
2700 Stuart Avenue
Richmond, VA 23220
(804) 359-3743

The Braille Circulating Library lends devotional, evangelical, doctrinal, and biographical books, Christian fiction, the Bible, and books for juveniles in braille, on talking book records, reel-to-reel and cassette tapes, and in large print. Catalogs of books, records and tapes are available from the Library. Services are free and worldwide.

Christian Record Braille Foundation, Inc. (CRBF)
4444 South 52nd Street
Lincoln, NE 68506
(402) 488-0981
(800) 228-4189

The Christian Record Braille Foundation (CRBF) provides services to visually and physically handicapped persons who cannot read normal print. Services include scholarships to blind and physically handicapped youth, glaucoma screening clinics, a camp for blind children, and Bible correspondence courses. Materials include talking magazines and tapes, cassettes, records, and large print books on a variety of subjects. CRBF maintains an extensive lending library of books on records, 7-inch reel tapes, cassettes, and in braille and large print. All materials are free.

Ephphatha Services for the Deaf and Blind (ES)
P.O. Box 713
Sioux Falls, SD 57101
(605) 339-0066

Ephphatha Services for the Deaf and Blind (ES) is a special service agency of the American Lutheran Church designed to stimulate member congregations to identify and serve handicapped individuals in their communities. ES maintains a Church registry of sensory impaired persons and has literature containing suggestions for identifying and locating sensory impaired individuals and integrating them into the Church community. ES offers religious counseling services and distributes religious periodicals on tape, cassette, and in braille. Ephphatha offers a free braille and tape transcription service.

Episcopal Guild for the Blind
157 Montague Street
Brooklyn, NY 11201
(212) 625-4886

The Guild provides blind or visually impaired individuals with the teachings and devotional literature of the Episcopal Church through braille and large type books, and cassette and disc recordings. The Guild also acts as an information center in areas pertinent to blindness, such as public and private resources and facilities, and assists blind persons and their families and friends in making application to appropriate facilities.

Gospel Association for the Blind, Inc.
P.O. Box 62
Del Ray Beach, FL 33444
(305) 395-0022

The Gospel Association for the Blind furnishes religious material in braille, talking books, and cassettes to blind individuals throughout the U.S. and 47 other countries. The Association conducts a summer camp for blind teenagers and adults, and provides temporary direct aid to newly blinded persons while directing them to more permanent sources of income, welfare, or rehabilitation. It also sponsors weekly religious radio broadcasts.

John Milton Society for the Blind
29 West 34th Street, 6th Floor
New York, NY 10001
(212) 736-4162

The John Milton Society for the Blind publishes Christian literature in braille, on records (talking books), and in large type on behalf of most Protestant denominations. The literature is intended for children and adults and is sent free to anyone who cannot read ordinary printed material. The Society gives small donations to church-related schools and homes for blind children.

**Lutheran Braille Evangelism Association
(LBEA)**
660 East Montana Avenue
St. Paul, MN 55106
(612) 772-1681

The Lutheran Braille Evangelism Association (LBEA) publishes and distributes Christian literature for blind and visually impaired persons. Bible materials, including the complete Bible, New Testament, and Psalms, are available in braille, cassettes, and large print. Devotional magazines are available in braille and large print. No blind person is denied materials because of inability to pay.

Lutheran Braille Workers, Inc. (LBW)
11735 Peach Tree Circle
Yucaipa, CA 92399
(714) 797-3093

The Lutheran Braille Workers (LBW) produce large print and braille religious (primarily Biblical) materials for free distribution to all who need them. Braille materials are produced in three grades of English braille and in 29 foreign language brailles.

Lutheran Library for the Blind
3558 South Jefferson Avenue
St. Louis, MO 63118
(314) 664-7000

The Lutheran Library for the Blind has a large collection of religious materials for the blind and visually impaired. Its materials (in braille, talking book form, tapes, and large print) are loaned throughout North America and some foreign countries. Catalogs are available from the Library, as is information about the services provided by other agencies for the blind. All Library services are free.

Ministries to the Deaf and Blind (MDB)
Division of Home Missions
General Council of Assemblies of God
1445 Boonville Avenue
Springfield, MO 65802
(417) 862-2781

Ministries to the Deaf and Blind (MDB) produces religious literature for blind and deaf persons and trains religious workers to carry out the ministry. Among MDB's materials are: pamphlets and Bible study manuals illustrated in sign language; books, pamphlets, and hymnals in braille and on cassette; and films and other audiovisual materials. Rental fees are charged for some materials; others are free or available on loan.

Ministry to the Deaf
Lutheran Church-Missouri Synod
500 North Broadway
St. Louis, MO 63102
(314) 231-6969

The Ministry to the Deaf provides a spiritual and social ministry to deaf and hearing handicapped persons in the U.S. and overseas. Its primary emphasis is on the profoundly deaf who are served through its 55 organized self-sustaining deaf churches and congregations. The Ministry trains volunteers and professionals, both hearing and deaf, for its ministry. Available materials include audiovisuals, brochures, and a newsletter. Statistical information related to the deaf and the families and teachers of the deaf in the Lutheran Church is maintained by the Ministry.

National Catholic Education Association
   (NCEA)
Special Education Department
One Dupont Circle
Sutie 350
Washington, DC 20036
(202) 293-5954

The Special Education Department of the NCEA serves as a clearinghouse of information on developments in legislation and in mainstreaming of handicapped children into regular classrooms. NCEA publishes the *Directory of Catholic Special Facilities and Programs in the United States for Handicapped Children and Adults*, bibliographies of research, and a newsletter. Users of the clearinghouse are Catholic schools and dioceses which provide special education services.

National Catholic Office of the Deaf
Trinity College
Washington, DC 20017
(202) 234-4154

The National Catholic Office of the Deaf provides teaching materials for religious education and organizes training programs for hearing impaired individuals, teachers, and parents. It organizes workshops which provide orientation and training in work with hearing impaired persons. Information relating to the religious education of the hearing impaired is available from the Office.

National Congress of Jewish Deaf (NCJD)
9102 Edmonston Court
Greenbelt, MD 20770

The National Congress of Jewish Deaf (NCJD) is a parent organization, advocating religious and cultural ideals and fellowship. NCJD conducts orientation seminars and workshops, assists in religious classes, supports a youth camp program, and provides religious publications. The Congress maintains an endowment fund and provides grants to tutor rabbis in sign language. A book of Jewish signs is being prepared for publication and will be available in early 1981.

Xavier Society for the Blind
154 East 23rd Street
New York, NY 10010
(212) 473-7800

The Xavier Society for the Blind publishes materials for visually impaired persons; textbooks for students and religious and devotional materials are priority items. The Society's collection of braille, large type, and taped books are available on loan through the mail. Catalogs of titles in each of the three forms are available on request.

SPORTS ORGANIZATIONS SERVING THE HANDICAPPED

American Athletic Association of the Deaf
3916 Lantern Drive
Silver Spring, MD 20902
(301) 942-4042

American Blind Bowling Association
150 N. Bellaire Avenue
Louisville, KY 40206
(502) 896-8039

American Wheelchair Bowling Association
224 N. Federal Highway, #109
Boynton Beach, FL 33435

Blind Outdoor Leisure Development (BOLD)
533 E. Main Street
Aspen, CO 81611
(303) 925-8922

Handicapped Sportspersons Association
  of Sacramento
3738 Walnut Avenue
Carmichael, CA 95608
(916) 484-2153

Indoor Sports Club
1145 Highland Street
Napoleon, OH 43545
(419) 592-5756

International Committee of the Silent Sports
Gallaudet College
Florida Avenue and Seventh St., N.E.
Washington, DC 20002
(202) 651-5114 (Voice or TTY)

National Foundation for Happy Horsemanship
  for the Handicapped
Box 462
Malvern, PA 19355
(215) 644-7414

National Handicapped Sports and
  Recreation Association
5672 S. Pierson Street
Littleton, CO 80123
(303) 978-0564

National Wheelchair Athletic Association
40-24 62nd Street
Woodside, NY 11377
(212) 898-0976

National Wheelchair Basketball Association
110 Seaton Center
University of Kentucky
Lexington, KY 40506
(606) 257-1623

North American Riding for the Handicapped
  Association, Inc.
P.O. Box 100
Ashburn, VA 22011
(703) 777-3540

United States Deaf Skiers Association
159 Davis Avenue
Hackensack, NJ 07601
Contact: Don Fields

Wheelchair Pilots Association
11018 102nd Avenue, N.
Largo, FL 33540
(813) 393-3131

NATIONAL DIRECTORIES OF SERVICES AND RESOURCES
FOR THE HANDICAPPED

American Annals of the Deaf (reference issue of journal): 1979, $6.50. American Annals of the Deaf, 5034 Wisconsin Avenue NW, Washington, DC 20016. Tel.: (202) 363-1327.

This reference issue, published annually in April, supplies information on programs and services for the deaf in the U.S., including educational, rehabilitational, social, and recreational listings. Most information is listed by state.

Directory: Cystic Fibrosis Centers for Diagnosis and Treatment of Cystic Fibrosis and Other Pediatric Pulmonary and Gastrointestinal Diseases: 1979, 250 pages, free. Cystic Fibrosis Foundation, 6000 Executive Boulevard, Suite 309, Rockville, MD 20852. Tel.: (301) 881-9130.

State listings with descriptive information on services of each center. Updated as needed, with no definite schedule.

Directory for Exceptional Children: 1978, 1300 pages, $25.00. Porter-Sargent Publishers Inc., 11 Beacon Street, Boston, MA 02108. Tel.: (617) 523-1670.

This directory lists schools, treatment centers, speech and hearing societies, state and private residential and day programs, etc. Descriptions of services are included. A new edition is expected to be available in 1980.

Directory of Agencies Serving the Visually Handicapped in the United States: 1978, 437 pages, $10.00. American Foundation for the Blind, Inc., 15 West 16th Street, New York, NY 10011. Tel.: (212) 620-2000.

State listings of educational, rehabilitation, and library services for the visually handicapped as well as organizations of national interest to the blind and those with low vision.

Directory of Education Facilities for the Learning Disabled: 1979-80, 59 pages, $1.00 plus $.50 postage. Association for Children with Learning Disabilities, 4156 Library Road, Pittsburgh, PA 15234. Tel.: (412) 341-1515.

State listing with descriptions of facilities. Updated annually.

Directory of Halfway Houses and Community Residences for the Mentally Ill: 1978, 38 pages, Pub. No. ADM 78-594, free. National Institute of Mental Health, Public Inquiries, 5600 Fishers Lane, Room 11A21, Rockville, MD 20857. Tel.: (301) 443-4515.

State listings of facilities with brief descriptions.

Directory of Hemophilia Treatment Centers: 1979, 62 pages, $2.00 plus postage (free to chapter members). National Hemophilia Foundation, 25 West 39th Street, New York, NY 10018. Tel.: (212) 869-9740.

State listings of treatment centers with brief descriptions of services. Updated annually.

Directory of National, Federal, and Local Sickle Cell Disease Programs: 1978, 30 pages, Pub. No. NIH 78-714, free. Sickle Cell Disease Branch, Division of Blood Diseases and Resources, National Heart, Lung and Blood Institute, Federal Building, Room 504, Bethesda, MD 20014. Tel.: (301) 496-6931.

State listings.

Directory of Organizations Interested in the Handicapped: 1980, 60 pages, $2—handicapped individuals or their families; $3—all others. People to People Committee for the Handicapped, 1522 K Street NW, Washington, DC 20005. Tel.: (202) 638-2487.

Lists and describes more than 200 national organizations that serve the handicapped as well as state vocational rehabilitation agencies, developmental disability programs, and employment security offices.

Guide to Epilepsy Services: 1978, 279 pages, free. Epilepsy Foundation of America, 1828 L Street NW, Suite 406, Washignton, DC 20036. Tel.: (202) 293-2930.

Lists and describes epilepsy clinics throughout the country as well as local chapters of the Foundation.

Membership Referral Roster: 1978, 70 pages, free. Academy of Dentistry for the Handicapped, 1726 Champa, Suite 422, Denver, CO 80202. Tel.: (303) 573-0264.

State listings of dentists and hygienists interested in improving the quality of dental care of the handicapped. Updated every two years.

National Association of Private Residential Facilities for the Mentally Retarded: Directory of Members: 1979, 40 pages, $15.00. National Association of Private Residential Facilities for the Mentally Retarded, 6269 Leesburg Pike, Falls Church, VA 22044. Tel.: (703) 536-3311.

State listings with brief descriptions of members' services. Updated every two years.

The 1978 Guide to Clinical Services in Speech-Language Pathology and Audiology: 1978, 191 pages, $8.00. American Speech-Language-Hearing Association, 10801 Rockville Pike, Rockville, MD 20852. Tel.: (301) 897-5700.

Contains profiles of clinical services and lists of private practitioners in speech and audiology. Also lists state resource personnel.

Research Directory of Rehabilitation Research and Training Centers: 1980, free to organizations in the rehabilitation field. National Institute of Handicapped Research, Department of Health, Education, and Welfare, Washington, DC 20201.

Covering fiscal year 1979, this directory contains abstracts of all research projects conducted by the Rehabilitation Services Administration's research and training centers. Updated annually.

Resource Directory of Handicapped Scientists: 1979, free. Project on the Handicapped in Science, Office of Opportunities in Science, American Association for the Advancement of Science, 1776 Massachusetts Avenue NW, Washington, DC 20036. Tel.: (202) 467-4497 (voice or TTY).

Lists more than 500 handicapped scientists available for consultation to educators, employers, and other professionals interested in making science education and science careers more accessible to the disabled.

Special Education Programs for Emotionally Disturbed Adolescents: A Directory of State Education Agency Services: 1978, 44 pages, $4.00. NASDSE, 1201 16th Street NW, Washington, DC 20036. Tel.: (202) 833-4193.

Results of a National Association of State Directors for Special Education survey, listing and describing services by state.

Special Education Programs for Severely Handicapped Students: A Directory of State Education Agency Services: 1979, 53 pages, $4.00. NASDSE, 1201 16th Street NW, Washington, DC 20036. Tel.: (202) 833-4193.

Annotated listings of services in special education for severely handicapped individuals, listed by state.

A Training and Resource Directory for Teachers Serving Handicapped Students K through 12: 1977, 213 pages, free. Office for Civil Rights, HEW, Room 5146, 330 Independence Avenue SW, Washington, DC 20201. Tel.: (202) 245-7504.

Lists national resource organizations, as well as state special education resources. Descriptive information is included.

National Directories That Include Services and
Resources of Importance to the Handicapped

Directory of Agencies: U.S. Voluntary, International Voluntary, Intergovernmental: 1978, 98 pages. $5.00 plus 10% for postage. National Association of Social Workers, 1425 H Street NW, Washington, DC 20005. Tel.: (202) 628-6800.

> Lists membership, purpose, and programs of more than 300 voluntary agencies that provide social work related services, including services for the handicapped.

Directory of Cancer Research Information Resources: 1979, 250 pages, Order Number PB293 187. $10.75, (North American Continent), double (foreign orders). National Technical Information Service, Subscription Department, Sills Building, 5285 Port Royal Road, Springfield, VA 22161.

> International in scope, this directory is designed to provide cancer researchers with a single-volume listing of available cancer information sources around the world. Covers more than 725 publications and information sources. Updated annually.

Directory of Community Health Centers: 1978, 15 pages, free. Program Services Branch, Bureau of Community Health Services, Room 7-08, 5600 Fishers Lane, Rockville, MD 20857. Tel.: (301) 443-3196.

> Regional list of community health centers that provide primary medical care, using a sliding fee schedule, to medically underserved populations including the handicapped.

Directory of Homemaker-Home Health Aide Service in the United States, Canada, Puerto Rico, and the Virgin Islands: 1977, 412 pages, $10.00. National Council for Homemaker-Home Health Aide Services, 67 Irving Place, New York, NY 10003. Tel.: (213) 674-4990.

> State listings of 3675 service units that provide home health aide services. A new edition is expected to be available in early 1980.

Directory of Information and Referral Services in the U.S. and Canada: 1978, 229 pages, $5.00 to members, $6.00 to nonmembers. Alliance of Information and Referral Services, PO Box 10705, Phoenix, AZ 85064. Tel.: (602) 263-7857.

> State listings of information and referral agencies that provide services to the handicapped and other populations. Updated every two years.

Encyclopedia of Associations: National Organizations of the U.S.: 1979, 1566 pages, $90.00. Gayle Research Co., Book Tower, Detroit, MI 48225.

> This comprehensive directory is a guide to national and international organizations and associations including trade, business, legal, government, educational, technical, health, and medical, etc. Pertinent descriptive information on each organization is included.

National Directory of Children and Youth Services: 1979, 538 pages, $39. CPR Directory Services Co., 1301 20th Street NW, Washington, DC 20036. Tel.: (202) 785-4061

> This directory includes more than 20,000 listings of public and private agencies throughout the country that serve children and youth. Updated annually.

National Directory of State Agencies: 1978-79, 679 pages, $55. plus $2.65 for postage. Information Resources Press, 1700 North Moore Street, Arlington, VA 22209. Tel.: (703) 558-8200.

> This directory contains lists of: agency functions, state government information phone numbers and addresses, agencies by state, agencies by function, and associations of state government officials.

The 1979 Directory of Federally Funded Community Mental Health Centers: 1979, 85 pages, Pub. No. ADM 79-258. single copies free. National Institute of Mental Health, Public Inquiries Section, Room 11A21, 5600 Fishers Lane, Rockville, MD 20857. Tel.: (301) 443-4513.

State listings.

Miscellaneous

International Telephone Directory of the Deaf: 1979, 132 pages, $5.00. Telecommunications for the Deaf, Inc., 814 Thayer Avenue, Silver Spring, MD 20910. Tel.: (301) 588-4605, voice; (301) 587-3006, TTY.

Lists TTY numbers of agencies and organizations that serve the deaf as well as individuals who are members of the organization. Updated annually.

International Directory of Access Guides: 1978-79, 24 pages, free Rehabilitation International, USA, 20 West 40th Street, New York, NY 10018. Tel.: (212) 869-9907.

Lists more than 325 cities that publish access guides for the elderly and handicapped. Updated annually.

U.S Rehabilitation Facilities Which Welcome Foreign and American Professional Visitors, 1979, 16 pages, $1.50 (US), free (abroad). Host Directory, Rehabilitation International, USA, 20 West 40th Street, New York, NY 10018. Tel.: (212) 869-0461.

Updated annually, the directory lists almost 300 facilities with basic descriptive information.

Directory of Information Resources for the Handicapped

ORGANIZATIONS AND FEDERAL AGENCIES

All Federal Agencies are asterisked for easy identification.

This is the alphabetical listing of all organizations and Federal agencies that appear in this DIRECTORY. The codes show the chapter where the organization or agency appears:

A = Advocacy, Consumer, Voluntary Health
I = Information/Data Banks
G = Federal Govt. Other Than Information Units
P = Professional and Trade Organizations
F = Facilities, Schools, Clinics
S = Service Organizations
AR = Appendix-Religious
AS = Appendix-Sports

HOW TO USE THE INDEX

The index is merely a guide to the organizations that might be relevant to an inquiry. It will put the user on the track of the national-level organizations that may be able to respond to his/her need. However, it **cannot substitute** for careful reading and screening of the abstracts in the directory for pertinence to one's query.

Every attempt was made to be brief and practical. The aim was to create useful entries, via index terms, to the organizations that could be helpful. For some organizations and some topics, this required indexing in more detail than others.

Index terms are primarily of two kinds: disorder terms (e.g., EPILEPSY) and non-disorder terms (e.g., EDUCATION, VOCATIONAL REHABILITATION, FUNDING, PROSTHETICS, VETERANS, and so on).

Disorder Terms

Approximately 102 terms have been used to describe specific disorders or general categories of disorders. If an organization covers most neurological disorders, it will appear under NEUROLOGICAL DIS-ORDERS but not under the many specific terms such as EPILEPSY, PARKINSON'S DISEASE, and the like. If you are looking for all organizations with information on epilepsy, you must look under EPILEPSY and also under the broader categories into which epilepsy would fit: NEUROLOGICAL DISORDERS and DEVELOPMENTAL DISABILITIES.

Information operations covering all or many aspects of a broad field like MEDICINE have been indexed only to this broad term, and no attempt has been made to index them to specific disorder or non-disorder terms.

Non-Disorder Terms

Organizations whose information covers subjects pertinent to all handicaps or to all physical handicaps are indexed by **non-disorder terms** such as EDUCATION, RECREATION, CAREERS, etc., but **not** by the 100 or more disorders which could conceivably be covered by that agency.

Our inability to define every term precisely and uniformly is handled by SEE ALSO references, which will alert you to related terms. When you seek information on a very precise and narrow subject, you will have to contact the organizations themselves to find out whether they cover your specific interest; the index will only have given you a solid lead, through the use of selected broad and specific terms.

Be sure to read the scope notes which accompany many of the terms. These notes give valuable information on areas covered or omitted by the terms.

INDEX

All Federal Agencies are asterisked for easy identification.

Organizations covering specific disorders are only listed under disorder terms.

Organizations covering specific disorders are only listed under disorder terms.

Organizations covering specific disorders are only listed under disorder terms.

Organizations covering specific disorders are only listed under disorder terms.

Organizations covering specific disorders are only listed under disorder terms.

Organizations covering specific disorders are only listed under disorder terms.

Organizations covering specific disorders are only listed under disorder terms.

Organizations covering specific disorders are only listed under disorder terms.

Organizations covering specific disorders are only listed under disorder terms.

Organizations covering specific disorders are only listed under disorder terms.

Page

Organizations covering specific disorders are only listed under disorder terms.

Organizations covering specific disorders are only listed under disorder terms.

Organizations covering specific disorders are only listed under disorder terms.

Organizations covering specific disorders are only listed under disorder terms.

Organizations covering specific disorders are only listed under disorder terms.

Organizations covering specific disorders are only listed under disorder terms.

Organizations covering specific disorders are only listed under disorder terms.

Organizations covering specific disorders are only listed under disorder terms.

Organizations covering specific disorders are only listed under disorder terms.

Organizations covering specific disorders are only listed under disorder terms.

Organizations covering specific disorders are only listed under disorder terms.

Organizations covering specific disorders are only listed under disorder terms.

Organizations covering specific disorders are only listed under disorder terms.

Organizations covering specific disorders are only listed under disorder terms.

Organizations covering specific disorders are only listed under disorder terms.

Organizations covering specific disorders are only listed under disorder terms.

Organizations covering specific disorders are only listed under disorder terms.

Organizations covering specific disorders are only listed under disorder terms.

Organizations covering specific disorders are only listed under disorder terms.

Organizations covering specific disorders are only listed under disorder terms.

Directory of Information Resources for the Handicapped

Organizations covering specific disorders are only listed under disorder terms.

Organizations covering specific disorders are only listed under disorder terms.

Organizations covering specific disorders are only listed under disorder terms.

Organizations covering specific disorders are only listed under disorder terms.

Organizations covering specific disorders are only listed under disorder terms.

Organizations covering specific disorders are only listed under disorder terms.

231

Organizations covering specific disorders are only listed under disorder terms.

Organizations covering specific disorders are only listed under disorder terms.

Organizations covering specific disorders are only listed under disorder terms.

Organizations covering specific disorders are only listed under disorder terms.

Organizations covering specific disorders are only listed under disorder terms.